Making it Real: a practical guide to experiential learning of communication skills

Jill Thistlethwaite
Associate Professor in Medical Education
Office of Teaching and Learning in Medicine
University of Sydney, Australia

and

George Ridgway
Learning Advisor
Teaching and Learning Department
James Cook University
Queensland, Australia

Foreword by

Jonathan Silverman

Radcliffe Publishing
Oxford • Seattle

Radcliffe Publishing Ltd
18 Marcham Road
Abingdon
Oxon OX14 1AA
United Kingdom

www.radcliffe-oxford.com
Electronic catalogue and worldwide online ordering facility.

British Library Cataloguing in Publication Data

A catalogue record for this book is available from the British Library.

ISBN-10 1 84619 022 3
ISBN-13 978 1 84619 022 3

Typeset by Lapiz Digital Services, Chennai
Printed and bound by TJ International Ltd, Padstow, Cornwall

Contents

Foreword

Communication skills teaching in medicine has come of age. Many skirmishes have now been won and, in the last five or six years, communication skills teaching and assessment have become accepted as central core components of the medical education landscape.

It has sometimes seemed a long hard campaign with no resolution in sight. Over the last 17 years that I have personally been involved in the field, it has often felt that communication skills, despite their obvious importance, were never going to be incorporated into the curriculum in any meaningful and sustained way and were even less likely to be established as a central component of the assessment of learners' clinical competence.

But suddenly, things have really taken off and it is gratifying that all the efforts expended by so many people have come together to enable the subject to achieve such a strategic position. The days seem to have passed of endlessly having to try to explain the importance of communication as a core clinical skill, the evidence base that communication skills can be taught effectively and are not simply learned by experience, the theoretical and research evidence that exists to guide what skills to teach and the body of work that demonstrates that communication skills can be effectively assessed. Communication skills and communication skills teaching are probably the most extensively researched of any aspect of medical education – I guess as a new kid on the curriculum it has had to try harder than everything else to justify its very existence.

There is still resistance in some quarters that needs to be carefully addressed but the subject has become well established in so many undergraduate and postgraduate settings that we have reached a new stage in the development of the field. What is needed now is practical help in enabling medical educators throughout the world to put in place teaching sessions and assessments without endlessly reinventing the wheel. This important book by Jill Thistlethwaite and George Ridgway does just that. As its central component, this manual of experiential learning provides a bank of ready-made simulated patient scenarios that will prove invaluable to anybody setting up a programme from scratch – here is a collection of scenarios with information for facilitators, participants and simulated patients and hints on how to run sessions on specific topics. And it is clearly not just for beginners – those already running established programs will also find it so useful to be able to turn to a resource of simulated patient scenarios when planning a new session. Interestingly, as one of its first and most important objectives, the recently formed UK Council of Communication Skills Teaching in Undergraduate Medical Education has established a password-protected website to share scenarios between schools because of this very need.

As an example of how invaluable this book will be, I have personally already found it helpful in developing our established communication curriculum at the University of Cambridge. We have recently extended our medical course by six months and in our final year wish to improve our teaching of communication between health professionals and to focus more heavily on handovers, telephone discussions and teamwork. And, lo and behold, here is a chapter which enables me to plagiarise without embarrassment several pre-written scenarios about both doctor-doctor communication and doctor-health professional situations. Perhaps the most impressive aspect of this new book are the chapters on communication between health professionals, formal interactions between professionals such as appraisal, disciplinary procedures and supervisor-student interactions and recent developments in communication skills training. Here the authors take the use of simulated patients into previously uncharted waters to the benefit of us all.

One area which this book does not tackle extensively is how to specifically train simulated patients in how real patients actually behave in the medical interview. Simulated patients may not appreciate the stereotyped behaviour patterns that, as research demonstrates, frequently occur between doctors and patients. They may for instance not appreciate that real patients often do not reveal all their symptoms or concerns in one go or question their doctor overtly about the areas that they do not understand. Each simulated patient role that the authors present expertly provides name, age, setting and medical background and also a first person description of the background information, expectations, ideas and concerns of the patient. But what is sometimes missing is the exact words in response to the interviewer's first open-ended question and how to respond to specific types of questions or approaches, what to divulge spontaneously and what not to with regard to open questions, screening questions and specific closed enquiries. Similarly, in the explanation and planning scenarios, it is not always clear how much the patient will ask their concerns and questions without explicit encouragement from the interviewer. This one addition would considerably help simulated patients adopt their roles more effectively.

This one quibble should not detract from the importance of this new volume. Now educators can turn to a practical source of expert guidance in setting up sessions utilising simulated patients. As the authors say, the scenarios can then be adapted to the specific setting of the educational experience, the group participants and their stage of expertise. Experiential work with simulated patients is the most effective way of improving learners' communication skills and enabling sustained change in behaviour, yet requires extensive effort on behalf of facilitators and programme directors – it is a methodology that is expensive in time, resources and money and the small group approach required does not reward even the large medical schools of today with any economy of size. Therefore, practical, thoughtful and well-considered help such as Thistlethwaite and Ridgway provide in this new book is worth its weight in gold and will help so many educators as they strive to introduce this approach to learning into medical curricula and assessments.

Jonathan Silverman
Associate Clinical Dean and Director of Communication Studies
School of Clinical Medicine
University of Cambridge
March 2006

Preface

Nearly 30 years ago when I was a medical student I was taught to take a history: a structured interrogation of the patient that was supposed to help me diagnose medical problems. That structure is still very familiar to me today and I use it as a framework for my interactions with patients. However it is only a framework, and 30 years of learning, practice, clinical and educational experience are still helping me fill the gaps. I watch as today's medical students try to make sense of the connections between what they learn in 'communication skills' and what they are expected to do on the wards, still 'taking a history'.

The traditional medical history often neglects the fundamentals of the patient's experience of health and illness and the effect these have on daily living. The clinician aims to manipulate the patient's story into a format recognised by other clinicians but perhaps not always recognised by the patient: everyday language becomes medical jargon.

Communication skills teaching is now a part of every medical school curriculum and also many health professionals' degree courses. At a postgraduate level, certainly in general practice training, we may refer to consultation skills. Communication and consultation skills also encompass much more than history taking. No health professional should now be put into a position of 'breaking bad news' without the opportunity of rehearsing this in a safe and supportive environment; likewise with dealing with aggression, working with interpreters and tackling poorly performing colleagues.

In some quarters there is still a feeling that such training is the domain of primary care or perhaps psychology/psychiatry. In the past we were concerned about how students and junior doctors communicated with patients. Now I have heard and read some senior clinicians saying we have gone too far and that our graduates are great communicators but their medical and particularly basic science knowledge is poor. They want a return to more didactic teaching to ground doctors in anatomy and physiology. We say why can't our doctors and health professionals do both: know their stuff and communicate?

Jill Thistlethwaite
George Ridgway
March 2006

About the authors

Jill Thistlethwaite is associate professor in medical education in the Office of Teaching and Learning in Medicine at the University of Sydney. She worked for many years as a GP in Yorkshire, where her interest in medical education led to her first becoming a GP trainer and then a GP course organiser in Calderdale. From 1996–2003 she was senior lecturer in community-based education at Leeds Medical School, where she ran the personal and professional development course unit. She has been involved in communication skills training since 1990. She gained her PhD in medical education on the subject of shared decision making from the University of Maastricht in 2003. Jill writes extensively in the medical press and is a fellow of the Society of Medical Writers.

George Ridgway has a PhD in biochemistry from the University of London and a postgraduate certificate in education. He worked as a science teacher in Rochdale and then became involved in communication skills teaching first as a simulated patient and then as a facilitator at Leeds University. Since moving to Australia in 2003 he has worked in communication skills training and as a learning advisor at James Cook University in Queensland. He is now a freelance educator.

Acknowledgements

We would like to thank all the simulated patients and facilitators we have worked with over the years in Calderdale, Leeds and Townsville. In particular Jill would like to acknowledge course administrator Liz Cockayne and community liaison officer Barry Ewart for helping make the PPD course a success. Jill would also like to acknowledge how much she has learnt from her patients.

Chapter 1

Introduction: the importance of communication skills

This chapter explores:

- how to use this book
- why teach communication skills?
- the communication skills literature relating to learning and teaching
- an overview of the use of simulated patients and their development
- the nature of experiential learning
- working with adult learners.

How to use this book

This book is a manual of experiential learning in relation to communication and consultation skills for health professionals. Most of the chapters begin with an outline of the topic and some background material. We give examples of how to run a session. There are a series of scenarios with information for facilitators, participants and the simulated patient (SP). The scenarios may be adapted depending on the group participants, stage of expertise and availability of SPs. Each topic and scenario has learning objectives or learning outcomes and points for facilitators. Suggestions are given for group discussion and debriefing. We refer to theoretical principles where appropriate.

Why communication skills training is important

As this book is more a practical manual than a reference text we will not go into detail about the evidence that health professionals need to be trained to communicate, and the problems that arise from poor communication. A search of the literature will reveal many studies relating to poor patient outcomes if good communication is not practised. However we will outline a few examples that may be used in introductory sessions for learners to highlight the importance of what they are about to study.

Health professional students, and in particular medical students, even early on in their training have a fear of being sued. It is important to stress to them that such litigation is often related to failure of some aspect of communication. For example, a book from the University of Michigan published in 2002 suggested that 80% of medical errors might be traced back to failure of communication.[1] A more recent report from the Picker Institute Europe, based on results of 15 national patient surveys in the UK between 1998 and 2005, found that 21% of outpatients and 26% of emergency department patients said staff didn't always listen carefully to what they were saying; 28% of inpatients said doctors talked in front of them; and 35% of mental health patients and 32% of outpatients said they did not receive clear explanations about risks and side-effects of medication. There had apparently been little improvement in any of these areas since previous surveys.[2] Also in the UK the Bristol Inquiry into the performance of paediatric heart surgeons showed that lack of communication was a factor in the poor outcomes for children undergoing surgery, including communication between different professionals caring for the patients.[3] Some of the recommendations relating to communication are shown in Box 1.1. In relation to adverse events and patient safety, Step 5 of the (UK) National Patient Safety Agency's (NPSA) *'Seven Steps to Patient Safety'* is 'Involve and communicate with patients and the public'.[4]

Box 1.1   Recommendations from the Bristol Inquiry[3]

- Involve patients/parents in decisions
- Keep patients/parents/carers informed
- Improve communication with patients/parents
- Provide patients and families with counselling and support
- Gain informed consent for all procedures and processes
- Elicit feedback from patients and listen to their views
- Be open and candid when adverse events occur

Research into the effects of good and bad communication is plentiful.[5] In summary, good communication leads to more accurate diagnosis, greater patient satisfaction, a greater likelihood that patients will adhere to treatment decisions, a reduction in stress and anxiety, better quality of life and an improvement in doctors' own wellbeing.

The communication skills literature

This book is not about the theory of communication skills or a major contribution to the educational literature, but rather it is a handbook of teaching and learning material arising from our experience as facilitators of experiential learning across all ranks, with an emphasis on communication and the doctor–patient consultation. We will also look at examples of communication outside the consulting room. Learning is experiential through the use of simulated patients (and simulated doctors, health professionals and students etc). References and guides to further reading are given for those readers interested in exploring theory in more depth.

Why simulated patients?

There are a number of ways to learn and teach communication and consultation skills (*see* Box 1.2). All have their advantages and disadvantages. In our opinion one of the most powerful methods for the learner is interacting in a safe environment with a SP. Reasons for this are given in Box 1.3. Howard Barrows at McMaster University in Ontario introduced the simulated patient technique in 1962, describing the development in a monograph published in 1971.[6] Since then, innovation and dissemination has led to increasing sophistication in the use of SPs in learning and assessing. However note that we now prefer to say 'working' with simulated patients rather than 'using' SPs; in the same way that we would work with real patients rather than use them (or indeed refer to them as clinical material). Such terminology is important as we wish SPs to be partners with clinicians in developing communication skills training and authentic scenarios that really do draw on patients' experiences rather than solely the clinicians' version of what happens in consultations.

Box 1.2   Ways of learning communication skills

- Reading communication skills books
- Didactic lectures with a list of skills and video examples
- Watching videos of someone else's consultations
- Observing a clinician interacting with a patient
- Being observed oneself with a patient and given feedback
- Being given feedback by a patient in a clinical setting
- Videoing oneself and watching the interaction alone or in a group with feedback
- Role-play
- Working with a simulated patient
- SP gives feedback

Box 1.3   Benefits of working with simulated patients

- Facilitator and learner have some control over environment
- It is possible to plan specific learning outcomes by use of scenarios unlike opportunistic consultations in real clinical settings
- Ability to stop consultation at learning points if patient/learner is distressed
- May rerun consultation to try different strategies
- Immediate feedback from patient
- Feedback from group
- Learners can practise difficult consultations without risk of upsetting real patients
- Scenarios may be developed in response to learner's needs

Experiential learning and working with adults

We learn communication skills best by observation and practice. While there is a role for didactic teaching of skills through lectures, the main learning sessions should be interactive with plenty of opportunities for 'doing' and feedback. Given that medical students should be adult learners, and qualified health professionals certainly are, we need to apply adult learning theory when planning sessions with SPs. Learning is best carried out in small groups.

Small-group work and learning with simulated patients is labour intensive. When planning communication skills sessions think how many tutors and SPs are available, how many rooms there are and what your budget is. The optimal size for a small group is between four and six students, but the rising number of students means that small groups often contain more than ten students. Every student should have the opportunity to interview a SP at least once, but this may not be possible every week.

The theory behind such small-group work is based on adult learning theory, also known as experiential learning, i.e. learning through experience. The experiential learning cycle of Kolb, derived from the earlier work of Lewin, is well known (*see* Figure 1.1).[7] This process of learning from observation and experience, via reflection and trying out new ways of doing things, is the perfect vehicle for learning communication skills. While a learner may move round the cycle in a workplace, the process is also possible within a more structured SP learning session. The observation and reflection is now no longer an individual process, but also involves the patient and the group members, adding value to skill development.[8]

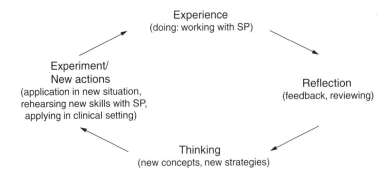

Figure 1.1 Kolb's experiential learning cycle in relation to working with simulated patients.

By observing and practising communication and consultation skills in small groups and with SPs, learners develop the tools they need to continue to develop in clinical settings. In such settings role models are important. We all learn from watching experts in action, we also learn what not to do, but only if we have a grounding in theory and practice in reflection. The old apprenticeship model of learning communication is not enough, neither is being thrown into the deep end and having to learn to communicate in difficult circumstances on the job. In clinical settings, learners are rarely observed and are even less likely to receive feedback, so experiential, classroom learning is vital for early skills development and also for skills consolidation in later years.

The development of expertise

Feedback and reflection are important components of experiential learning and help learners develop expertise. The competency cycle (*see* Figure 1.2) is a useful way of showing learners the importance of feedback and how working with SPs will enhance their skills in communication.[9] While many students starting their health professional studies will feel that they already have some competence in communication (and this is of course true), they do not know what they do not know about communicating with patients. They are unconsciously incompetent. By observing a consultation they realise that there are certain skills they need to work within their new environment (consciously incompetent). By interacting with SPs, being given feedback by the SPs and facilitators, and reflecting on their own performance, they develop conscious competence. Eventually, hopefully, they become experts (though there is always room for improvement through being observed and working with SPs once qualified).

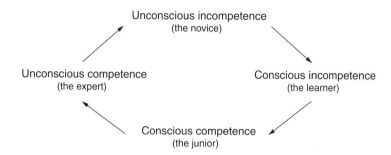

Figure 1.2 The competency cycle.

The introductory session

At the beginning of an undergraduate course on communication skills, a lecture may be a useful way of conveying a certain amount of knowledge information to a large group of people. This is particularly appropriate in medical schools where year groups now often number over 200 students and may reach 300. The possible content of an introductory lecture prior to experiential small-group sessions is shown in Box 1.4.

Box 1.4   An introduction to communication skills

- Introduction to communication skills staff
- Why communication is important for health professionals
- The evidence for good communication
- What happens when communication goes wrong
- Ways of learning communication
- Methods of giving feedback
- Playing a video of a doctor consulting with a patient
- The feedback process on the video clip
- Further reading
- What happens next

Showing a real consultation to year 1 students can be the highlight of the session. Obviously patient consent is needed. At this stage the consultation should be fairly typical of a doctor's working day: it should include material for discussion. The optimum video will be of one of the doctors involved in the lecture, as feedback can be given directly to that doctor, mirroring what will happen in the small-group sessions later on. In this way the doctor acts as a role model, being amenable and indeed eager for feedback on his/her performance. Therefore the consultation should not be picked as a 'good' consultation or a 'poor' consultation. Unless the patient is available as well, the lecturer should point out that the feedback does lack the patient's voice, but that in the coming work with SPs, the patient's voice is a powerful component in the learning process.

If a video is not available, or as an alternative, one of the lecturers may interview a SP in the lecture theatre and then run through the feedback process. Now there is a chance to receive patient feedback. Attention needs to be paid to sound levels, and if possible roving microphones should be used. While this modelling of a session is helpful, we think that a video of a real consultation is preferable as the students see what they will be doing in a few years' time, and begin to understand the importance of doctors continually reviewing their work and performance.

Summary

The introduction to communication/consultations skills learning is an important part of any skills course. Course organisers should stress the theoretical basis of learning and the importance of the topic. However, learners are keen to move onto practical sessions; too much didactic teaching is likely to lose their interest. Theory can be further highlighted during experiential learning sessions.

References

1 Rosenthal MM, Sutcliffe KM (eds). *Medical error: what do we know? What do we do?* New Jersey: Jossey-Bass, 2001.

2 The Picker Institute. *Is the NHS getting better or worse?* www.pickereurope.org (accessed 3 February 2006).

3 Bristol Royal Infirmary Inquiry. *Learning from Bristol: the report of the public inquiry into children's heart surgery at the Bristol Royal Infirmary 1984–1995.* CM5207. London: Stationery Office, 2001. www.bristol-inquiry.org.uk/ (accessed 3 February 2006).

4 National Patient Safety Agency. *Seven Steps to Patient Safety. The full reference guide.* www.npsa.nhs.uk/sevensteps (accessed 3 February 2006).

5 Silverman J, Kurtz S and Draper J. *Skills for Communicating with Patients.* Oxford: Radcliffe Medical Press, 2004.

6 Barrows HS. *Simulated Patients (Programmed Patients). The development and use of a new technique in medical education.* Illinois: Charles C Thomas, 1971.

7 Kolb DA. The process of experiential learning. In: Thorpe M, Edwards R and Hanson A (eds). *Culture and Processes of Adult Learning.* London: Routledge. 1993; 138–56.

8 Elwyn G, Greenhalgh T and Macfarlane F. *Groups. A guide to small group work in healthcare, management and research.* Oxford: Radcliffe Medical Press, 2001.

9 Bayley H, Chambers R and Donovan C. *The Good Mentoring Toolkit for Healthcare.* Oxford: Radcliffe Medical Press, 2004.

Chapter 2

A practical guide to working with simulated patients and as a simulated patient

This chapter explores:

- the recruitment and training of simulated patients
- the competencies that simulated patients require
- simulated patients working with facilitators
- achieving realism in roles
- developing scenarios
- how to ensure a safe learning environment
- caring for simulated patients.

A simulated patient (SP) is now a trained and valuable member of the health professional education team. As such, SPs require training and professional development, moving from being role-players in simple interactions to educators and facilitators who are able to give feedback and assess learners.

Recruitment of simulated patients

The success of any learning experience using simulated patients depends to a great extent on the calibre and skills of the simulated patients. While SPs are predominantly acting or role-playing, they need to bring emotional intelligence to their performance. Moreover the best SPs have the ability to understand the way their character is thinking and feeling in a holistic manner about the doctor–patient interaction in which they are engaged. To develop this understanding they might draw on their own experience as patients; conversations with friends who are or have been patients; conversations with healthcare professionals; reading general articles (newspapers, magazines); listening to public discourse about patient issues; talking to people such as prisoners, substance misusers or patients who have had a particular consultation type with a doctor e.g. for abortion or depression. When recruiting SPs we are looking for people who have a continued interest in improving the simulations with which they are involved.

Almost all of the people recruited to be simulated patients will have had experience of seeing a doctor or other health professional; almost all will have experience of being ill, perhaps seriously. Professional actors often immerse themselves in a role prior to performance. For example the Stanislavsky school of method acting (*see* Box 2.1) recommends actors living as their characters in order to gain insight into the emotions and behaviour they need to portray. SPs do not need to subscribe to the method acting way, as they already know what it feels like to consult as themselves. However the skill required in the learning situation is using those experiences to inform their roles, to act and react as their character. The SP should ask the question: 'what would this patient do in this situation?' not 'what would I do in this situation?' A timid simulated character will not challenge a doctor who uses jargon for example, while the real person might.

Box 2.1 Stanislavsky and method acting[1]

Konstantin Stanislavsky (1863–1938) was an actor and founder of the Moscow Art Theatre. His method acting system helped actors develop realistic characters, through the use of their emotion memory helping them portray a character's emotions as naturally as possible. The emotion memory involved actors thinking about a moment in their own lives when they had experienced the emotion of their character, and replaying it. Actors also have to analyse their character's motivation, rather than rely on the script to dictate their performance.

SPs do not need to have acting experience, though many are recruited from amateur dramatics societies or acting colleges. Resting professional actors are also a useful source, though they are likely to disappear at fairly short notice if they get a better offer of work. On the other hand, in big cities income from SP work can help develop an acting career in terms of skill development (giving feedback to a group or a director is valuable) and obtaining a regular income. Within a university setting postgraduate students are often willing to be SPs, certainly if they are paid. Advertising at local postgraduate medical education centres may attract part-time health professionals or practice staff, and indeed it is worth asking general practitioners (GPs) to discuss the vacancies with their receptionists and secretaries, as ancillary staff may be quite keen to become involved.

It is possible to advertise for SPs in the local press, but people coming without a personal recommendation from a reliable source will need vetting. As training sessions may involve discussion of roles based on real patient encounters it is important that recruited SPs are able to accept that doctors are not gods. There is no real issue of breaching confidentiality because no personal details concerning a consultation are ever revealed.

Potential SPs should be vetted for personal issues with health professionals. While it is acceptable that SPs would want to help students and qualified professionals improve their communication skills, because of their own or family's experiences of illness, it is important that this motive is not inappropriately applied. An SP's desire to participate in roles might be linked to negative feelings or bitterness toward all doctors. The expression of such emotions in sessions, particularly those involving junior students, can be very destructive and may jeopardise any learning experience. In any event a person with a vendetta against doctors for real or imagined negligence may not be able to give positive feedback. Before the preliminary training session all potential SPs should have an interview with one or more of the organising team. As all feelings may not be expressed fully in interviews, new SPs need to be monitored for adverse comments likely to upset learners. This is a strong argument for certificated training of SPs.

Training of simulated patients

There are many different levels on which an SP may work (*see* Box 2.2). Where an individual starts depends on their background, previous experience of educational activities, and ability. Some form of assessment of the potential SP is therefore needed. A suggested outline for a preliminary training session is shown in Box 2.3, with possible tasks for trios in Box 2.4. In a trio, two people role-play according to the activity outlined, and the third person observes. The session will need to be adapted depending on numbers. The session should be run by an experienced facilitator and include a number of trained SPs.

The activities are such that potential SPs will be able to gauge their ability and comfort in role-playing, have experience of giving feedback as observers and role-players and will rehearse atypical learning sessions. Facilitators will also be able to evaluate these competencies in the potential SP and watch for any 'personal baggage' that might interfere with teaching and learning.

The novice SP can gradually take on more responsibility using a typical 360° feedback, i.e. inviting comments on the SP's performance from the SP, others SPs, facilitators and learners.

Box 2.2   Different levels at which an SP works

- Observes a well-developed role given by an experienced SP and hears feedback elicited by an experienced facilitator × 3 different roles
- Role-plays a well-developed role; does not give feedback (may be taped and played back without SP being present)
- Role-plays a well-developed role; gives feedback out of role in facilitator-led session
- Role-plays a well-developed role; gives feedback in role in facilitator-led session
- Gives feedback in and out of role and can change the feedback mode to suit the desired learning outcome
- Role-plays a well-developed role for an examination; does not mark candidate, only observer/assessor marks
- Role-plays a well-developed role for an examination; marks simulated candidate only in relation to communication skills marks compared with experienced counterpart
- Role-plays a well-developed role for an examination; marks candidate on content using pro-forma and communication skills, no other observer/assessor present
- Ability to facilitate a small group is developed in a similar incremental manner
- Role-plays and can act as a facilitator of a small group
- As a facilitator builds roles during educational session from material supplied by participants

---

Box 2.3   Suggested initial training session

- Introductions: names, background, previous experience, why interested in this kind of work
- Definition of the aims or outcomes for the session

Continued

- Outline of the session
- Brief introduction to the world of the SP and the types of educational sessions that this particular group will be involved with, including the nature and purpose of communication/consultation skills training
- Brief introduction to ways of giving feedback
- Example of a consultation or learning activity involving an SP (one of the trained SPs will do this)
- Mirror the activity of a 'real session' by asking the trainee SPs to give feedback both to the SP and the interviewer
- Facilitated discussion on the content and process of the interview just watched
- Discussion of participants' ideas and concerns in playing roles themselves
- Break large group into trios and perform role-playing exercise: one person as interviewer, one person as interviewee, one as observer (this could be one of the experienced SPs present). Run role-play for 5–10 minutes and ask observer to give feedback
- In a large group discuss how this went: what went well, what was difficult
- Preliminary exploration of what makes a good interview: introduction, types of questions etc
- General discussion on role-playing, how to get into role, different types of roles
- Wrap-up: explore if any participant feels uncomfortable with what they are learning to do, answer any questions
- Speak to individuals if any concerns have been raised

Box 2.4   Trios for early training

1   A is a journalist who works for the local paper. He/she is to interview B about the new restaurant B opened a month ago: what sort of food does it serve, opening times, ambience etc.
2   A is interviewing B who has applied for a job as a drama teacher at the local secondary school. A will need to ask B about previous experience, teaching philosophy and what activities he/she proposes that the school puts on.
3   A is the triage nurse at the local hospital emergency department. A needs to assess the urgency of B's ankle injury, how it happened, what hurts etc.

Competencies for simulated patients

SPs give feedback in role and/or out of role. To do this they must have some understanding of the basics of the nature of medical interviewing and the nature of good communication skills. They need to know the 'jargon' of communication but, of course, they are not being trained to conduct medical consultations. Too much theory may hinder their feedback as patients. Working over time with students and health professionals who are learning and developing their communication skills means that SPs do absorb a tremendous amount of knowledge relating to professional–patient interactions. Quality assurance of the SPs' performance should be made regularly to ensure that the essence of their working as the patient's voice is not lost. Further training is best carried out under the apprenticeship model, in which novice SPs sit in with skilled SPs during educational sessions and watch how they work, with a debriefing session at the end in order to discuss what was seen and learnt. Once novice SPs start working themselves they should be paired up with an experienced facilitator to begin with. Training for examinations is also necessary to ensure reliability and fairness of marking. Competencies for SPs are listed in Box 2.5 starting with the basic and moving down to advanced competenecies.

Box 2.5   Competencies for SPs

- Acting a role
- Responding to an interviewer in character: how would this patient react to such a question?
- Showing emotion as appropriate
- Knowledge of communication skills language: open and closed questions, summarising, empathy, body language
- Knowledge of the purpose and basic outline of a medical interview
- Giving constructive feedback out of role
- Giving constructive feedback in role
- Developing new roles
- Staying faithful to a role in an examination situation
- Marking reliably

Authenticity in the patient role

The simulated patient roles should be as authentic as possible. There are various ways to achieve this. However the interactions are simulated and will always have some artificiality due to location, timing, observation or breaking down encounters into smaller chunks to match particular learning outcomes.

Developing scenarios

For certain situations the educator will completely write a scenario with the intention of introducing learners to a particular experience or in order to facilitate them developing specific skills such as listening, explaining or dealing with aggression. However these scenarios should be checked and the question asked: is this a likely interaction and development of character? Once written, the SPs chosen to work with the scenarios should be asked for their opinion as to the authenticity of the role. Do they feel comfortable with the way they are asked to respond? How do they feel the character would react to certain questions? For examinations it is important that the roles are standardised and all SPs react the same way to the same line of questioning and interaction. In teaching sessions the SPs have some flexibility to develop their role the way their interpretation of the character moves them.

Basing scenarios on real patients

Doctors and health professionals are also telling stories about their patient encounters (with no patient names mentioned). These are interesting to them because the patient has affected them in some way, because the interaction did not go the way expected, because there were difficulties or surprises. These stories are the raw material for SP scenarios and are more authentic because they are based on reality. However they still only give the viewpoint of the professional, and again the SP may be able to offer different insights into patient behaviour from the perspective of being a patient.

Often scenarios are based on an amalgam of patients, and these have to be checked carefully for authenticity. Care also needs to be taken that patients may not be identified from these roles: some aspects of the story may need to be changed.

Basing scenarios on videotapes of real consultations

This is a technique used to develop scenarios for important assessments in order to have validity. The SP works with a videotape of the patient and opens the interaction with the doctor with the same words that the real patient has used. The SP will respond as the real patient did if the doctor uses similar questions or explanations. However the SP needs to feel how the patient would react if the doctor interacts in a completely different way than the one taped. The real patients need to give informed written consent for their consultations to be used in this way (and consent to be videotaped). Again, once the patient has been taped, the patient voice is lost as the SP and educators work on the role together (though the patient could be invited to be part of this process).

The patient voice for developing scenarios

Groups of real patients working with simulated patients develop authentic roles based on their stories, and work through the many different ways that they could unfold with different professionals. This allows real patient ideas and concerns to be discussed and written into the scenarios. It also involves patients in deciding what aspects of communication are important for learners to develop. Self-help groups may wish to be involved in discussing their experiences, their symptoms, their concerns and the impact of any treatment they have received.

Achieving realism in roles: a personal insight

I have simulated 25 different patients for experiential learning group work, ranging from the painfully shy to the aggressively demanding. I have played hetero- and homosexual roles and those in low and high socio-economic groups. I prepare for roles mentally so that I behave like the character; physically so that I look like the character; and emotionally so that I feel like the character. I modify my accent to speak with received or regional pronunciation, although I would not risk credibility in order to achieve a particular accent.

I also dress in a manner that is consistent, if stereotypical, with a specific patient. For example if I am a substance abuser, I wear tracksuit bottoms, a dirty white T-shirt, off-white socks, old trainers and a hooded top or a nylon sports jacket. As a homeless patient, chocolate is excellent for 'dirt' or worse on light-coloured tops. A worker in the building industry wears denims, a shirt, and scuffed boots with concrete splashes on them and an outdoor coat. I keep my hair cut short for an aggressive look; this is easily counterbalanced for a calmer role by smiling. Before playing certain scenarios, real-life gardening in the rose bushes scratches my arms and can help me appear just like a gardener complete with soil under my nails or someone much more sinister if I am looking angry. Of course both of these examples are stereotypes, but this is what I mean by looking the part.

Such preparation is not always possible. A female may play a male role and vice versa. A young man may become an aged grandfather. However, if and when possible it creates authenticity if the SP matches the role and dresses for the part.

I might have been given a role several days or even weeks in advance. I would have read a scenario – a short history of my character. This contains details of my medical and social background. I would be free to add to it where necessary. I would start behaving in role before I entered the teaching room.

Some roles need an emotional charge for them to be realistic. To achieve this I recall real-life emotions and feel them during the scenario. Anger is quite easy to do, tears much less so. If my character would have broken down I need to be able to do the same, even though it is for a different reason. To do this I recall how I felt when my mother was very ill. Other stimuli are shown in Table 2.1.

Table 2.1   Emotional stimuli

Feeling in role	Stimulus
Anger	Driving on the M62 on a bad day
Aggression	Particular moments playing football
Depression	When my best friend died
Stress	Working in a poorly run department
Feeling physically ill	A real episode of personal ill-health
Feeling mentally ill	When I have felt not in control
Confrontational	Challenging a builder's bad work

I try to match emotions I have actually felt to kick-start those my character may feel. Sometimes the emotional depth of the simulated role is so deep that I have carried on with the character hours after coming out of role. This happens to me particularly with aggressive and emotional roles. My acting colleagues agree that it can be difficult to let go of a character, but they have their own personal 'roles that cling'. After a particularly strong role has been played, SPs like to be brought out more thoroughly and debriefed for example by a group hug, song, recited poem, or hand-holding. Goodness knows what mishaps this helps to prevent.

SPs may come from all areas of society. They may have disabilities, be from different cultural backgrounds from the majority of the learners or have chronic diseases that affect their communication. However their roles do not need to be based around these attributes. A patient with a disability may see a doctor for problems not specifically related to the disability. The disability obviously has some effects on the patients but the doctor has to move beyond what might be obvious and have an open mind as to the patient's ideas, concerns and expectations. Similarly an SP with a disability does not need to play a role in which the disability is the main focus. However the experience of SPs from diverse backgrounds can inform the development of roles, either for themselves or other SPs.

Working with facilitators

The best facilitators I have worked with seem to talk the least during the learning session, allowing the simulated patient, the learner and group members to talk and be heard. Good facilitators use the skills of the whole group to discuss points such as what the learner did well, what the learner could do differently and what reactions are apparent in the simulation. The simulated patient sessions in which I have participated have always included a facilitator. In role I can see and hear only the learner. However I 'allow' the facilitator to give broad instructions such as to play a role out for the full length of the interview, to allow a new interviewer to take over and to replay a section of the interview. During feedback the facilitator may also ask me to explain why I showed a specific reaction or feeling, to answer questions from the group, to say what went well and what could be done differently. The facilitator also informs me when to come out of role.

Even while I am in role I am prepared to take an instruction from the facilitator. I respond the way my role suggests I would. If a pause is required, as one character I might stare at the floor keeping the slight shake in my right hand going. A different patient bites his nails and clenches his teeth. If asked to leave the room, I do so in role! This means anything from slithering out to storming off with an expletive.

On occasion a learner has tried to pull me out of character during a simulated patient exercise and this has happened to other SPs. We have agreed that the best response to a challenge is a confused look and to repeat the last few words of the challenger prefaced with:

'What do you mean that I should . . .'?

For example:

- '. . . tell you my fears concerns and expectations as it's only a game?'
- '. . . come out of role as I am only pretending?'
- '. . . tell you what my hidden problem is?'
- '. . . explain to you whether you have passed the examination or not?'.

Any serious attempt to challenge the simulation should be reported to a facilitator.

On the other hand an SP should never risk a complaint against them and the team they belong to by offering help to selected interviewers. This can happen in group experiential learning programmes and it is not just closed summative examination conditions that allow collusion. In the former an SP may be tempted to give a particular learner information that has not been suggested by the interviewer's questioning. This should be picked up by other participants, particularly the facilitator, and commented on openly to produce the desired change in the erring SP.

In an examination-based setting, the marks of other SP roles can be compared and an unusual grading can be checked and the SP asked to provide comment.

An SP who has had a glass or two of wine jeopardises a whole evening's work if a single candidate's complaint is upheld. Other participants will notice this and will lose faith in the method, and they will not wish to pursue this learning style. In other words one unprincipled or inconsiderate SP can cause a lot of damage.

Simulated patient development

Good SPs will reflect on their roles and try to improve and develop their skills. Box 2.6 contains the sorts of questions that SPs may ask themselves and others to help refine their roles following a learning session.

Box 2.6   Refining the role

- Did I introduce myself as the patient might do?
- Are my symptoms correct?
- Is my patient knowledge okay or have I been listening to doctors too much?
- Do I follow the consultation in a patient like way i.e. *not* playing cat and mouse?
- Did I collude with the interviewer – was information unrealistically easy or difficult to obtain?
- Can anyone see or recall aspects of a real patient from what they have just experienced?
- Would learners pass on to me any tips related to the role they have just shared?

Payment for SPs

In our opinion SPs should be paid for the work they do. They are expected to work at a high standard, respect confidentiality and be reliable. The days of volunteer patients should be long gone (though this argument is debatable when applied to 'real' patients, who are often keen to be involved in helping students – in these cases it may be appropriate only to remunerate for expenses). SPs may also be involved in high-stakes examinations, during which their marks contribute to whether a candidate passes or fails. Such judgements should be recognised for the skill they require and payment be made at a suitable level.

Different institutions pay different amounts. The amounts may be on a scale commensurate with experience and the nature of the educational activity. SPs are usually paid on a casual basis for the work they do rather than being employed on a part- or full-time contract. For university work, demand for SPs may be higher at certain times of the academic year. Certainly a busy time is during clinical examinations. Whether SPs should be paid for training is a difficult question. Training is an integral part of the development of a good SP resource and if it is mandatory it should be financed. However a preliminary session to establish whether new recruits are suitable for the work may perhaps be run on an expenses-only basis.

When setting up a bank of simulated patients it is important that there is adequate money to cover costs and that the responsibilities of employers are recognised.

Caring for simulated patients

There has been very little research so far of the effects on people who work as simulated patients. Such effects might be expected to include difficulties when they need to consult a health professional as a 'real patient', and stress relating to the roles they play and an inability to come out of role when they have been playing a patient with a distressing condition. Anecdotally, some SPs have told us that they are often assessing the consulting skills of their own doctors and have to restrain themselves from giving feedback. From the small number of published studies on this topic, the general findings seem to suggest that the advantages to the SPs outweigh any disadvantages.[2] As mentioned earlier in the chapter, recruitment, training, good facilitation and the provision of a safe learning environment are important. There also needs to be adequate time for SPs to de-role and de-brief, and to discuss any emotional problems they might have encountered during a role at the end of a learning session.

Summary

Simulated patients require training and development to realise their full potential as educators in relation to communication and consultation skills. As SPs do become more skilled then institutions need to consider the levels of payment for SPs, particularly in recognition of their important role in assessment.

References

1 www.en.wikipedia.org/wiki/Konstantin_Stanislavsky (accessed 3 February 2006).
2 Spencer J, Dales J. Meeting the needs of simulated patients and caring for the person behind them. *Med Educ.* 2006; **40:** 3–5.

Chapter 3

A practical guide to individual sessions

This chapter explores:

- how to plan a learning session
- learning objectives and learning outcomes
- giving feedback
- choosing scenarios
- examples of sessions for different levels of participants
- setting objectives
- goldfish bowl versus video
- a communication/consultation skills curriculum
- evaluation.

This chapter provides a template for a generic educational session involving some form of simulation. The simulator may be a simulated patient, simulated student, simulated doctor etc, or a combination of the above. As the most common sessions involve simulated patients we will concentrate on a learning experience using SPs, but also give brief examples of sessions with other simulators.

Planning the session

When asked to run any educational session certain questions need to be answered in order to plan the input (*see* Box 3.1). If the group hasn't worked together before, more time will be needed for introductions. If none of the participants have worked with SPs before, more time will be needed for explaining working methods. The institution or convenor may set the learning objectives or outcomes, or they may be the responsibility of the educator running the session. With certain groups, particularly more senior health professionals, the group may set additional outcomes at the beginning of the session.

What the session sets out to do in terms of participant learning may be classified as either learning objectives or learning outcomes. In broad terms, objectives are written in terms of what the student will achieve, whereas outcomes are what the student will have achieved by the end of the activity. The outcome will be a new skill and/or new knowledge that will ultimately improve patient care.

Objectives and outcomes both communicate to the learner what is to be taught and hopefully learnt and what is required of the learner, and give some idea of the type and extent of the activity that will be engaged in to achieve this. In particular for students they will also want to know how they will be assessed, and any assessment of their new skills and knowledge should be derived from the specific objectives or outcomes that have been defined.

Box 3.1 Questions to be answered when planning a session

- Who will be attending the session: who will be the learners (e.g. medical students (what year?), GP registrars, specialists, health professionals, mixed inter-professional group etc)?
- How many will there be?
- How long will the activity last? Is it a one-off session or a series of sessions?
- What are the objectives or learning outcomes for the session? Who will set these?
- What do the participants already know about this topic?
- How does this session/do these sessions fit into the participants' course of study/ongoing education?
- Are there any particular scenarios that are needed?
- Have the participants any experience of working with SPs?
- Have the participants learnt together before? (Are they in already-formed groups?)
- What is the budget for the activity?
- What room(s) are available? How big are they?
- What other resources are needed and available (e.g. flipcharts, projector etc)?
- Has the session(s) already be named and/or advertised?
- Do we know what the participants are expecting?
- How will the session be evaluated? Who is responsible for this? Who wants the results of the evaluation (e.g. facilitator, course organiser, institution)?

The recent trend is to state learning outcomes rather than objectives, concentrating on the product rather than the process. In this book we will use both methods, as they are equally valid: the important educational issue is that learners know what is expected of them. At the end of a learning session the objectives/outcomes should be revisited to ensure that they have been covered. They may not have been fully achieved at this point, as learning should be consolidated by practice following the activity.

Giving feedback

One of the more widely used methods of giving feedback is the so-called 'Pendleton's rules'. These were first described by Pendleton and colleagues in their 1984 book *The Consultation*.[1] For example, at the end of an activity where a learner has interviewed a 'patient' (during role-play, a simulated patient, a real patient on a video etc), the learner is first asked to comment on what was done well. If the patient is present, the patient is then asked what was done well. Then the rest of the learning group and finally the facilitator comment on what was done well. The process is then repeated with participants commenting in the same order on what could be done differently to improve communication and/or the outcome of the consultation. In the 2003 second edition of *The Consultation*, Pendleton and colleagues responded to criticism of the rigidity of this approach by writing that these were never meant to be rules, but rather guidelines.[2]

These guidelines and method of feedback are extremely useful when first introducing students to giving and receiving feedback, as they know exactly what to expect. Students are reminded of the need to evaluate their own performance positively and to give concrete examples of how they would do things differently if asked to repeat an interaction. However for participants who are more familiar with experiential work, giving feedback should be adapted to their needs. In particular interviewers may be asked what it is they want the observers to focus on during their SP interaction and what they would most value feedback about.

Constructive feedback involves giving concrete examples of what the learner did, and should be non-judgemental. Good feedback should also invite the learner to reflect on his/her performance rather than spoon-feeding suggestions as to how things may be done differently. Rather than saying 'you really upset the patient that time', a more constructive approach would be 'the patient was upset, what do you think happened to upset her?'. Once the learner has given an opinion as to the cause of this emotion, the reason should be checked with the SP, as the interpretation of both the learner and the facilitator may not be completely accurate. Feedback to more senior participants should be challenging, without being threatening. There is no point in not drawing attention to poor communication skills if the learner him or herself does not pick these up.

Choosing scenarios

This will depend on two things: the objectives or learning outcomes of the session and the availability of SPs. It is of course much easier to use tried and tested scenarios and SPs experienced in those roles. However it may be necessary to develop new roles or adapt old ones to fit the needs of the participants and the anticipated outcomes. Certain roles may need to be played at different levels of intricacy depending on the experience of the learners. First year medical students will not be able to elicit a complicated medical history in a logical way, but may be able to elicit a patient's story without a lot of medical details. With new roles you must decide whether your chosen SPs need a training session prior to the activity. A training session may also be needed if the SPs have not worked with this particular type of participant before. Can this be budgeted for? Experienced SPs may be able to develop a role from an outline themselves, and training may not be needed, though the facilitator and SPs should meet prior to the start of the session to ensure that all are confident about their input.

The overall length of the session, and the number and seniority of the learners will affect the number of scenarios needed. First year medical students will probably only need to interact with an SP during a first attempt for up to ten minutes maximum, while a doctor 'breaking bad news' may require 15 to 20 minutes. Do you want all participants to have a chance to interview? Or is it acceptable for only one or two to be involved? Again this affects the number of roles and SPs needed.

Scenarios involving physical examinations

The aim of working with simulated patients is to develop and improve communication and consultation skills. Obviously doctor–patient and health professional–patient interactions often necessitate a physical examination of the patient. Except in certain circumstances we would not expect a patient to be examined. If the scenario requires an examination or the interviewer wishes to carry out an examination, the best way to proceed is to have the results of any examination written on a card that the SP can hand to the interviewer at the appropriate moment. Sometimes, and particularly in examinations when the results of the examination may have a bearing on what happens next, an SP may need more than one card with different systems on each (*see* Box 3.2 for an example). Participants in the learning sessions need to be aware of what to do when they wish to examine: they should be advised to say 'I would like to examine your abdomen' for example, and then the patient hands them the appropriate findings. Of course the interviewer should always ask to examine the patient and explain why this is so in a real consultation. The only difference with the simulation is that the actual examination is not carried out. If the scenario is only to be played once or twice in a session the SP may agree to have his/her throat examined or blood pressure taken.

Box 3.2   Example of examination cards

SP complains of headaches to doctor who elicits the history. Doctor asks to take patient's blood pressure. Is handed card that reads:

Pulse 76 regular, BP sitting 132/78.

Doctor states that he/she will examine the patient's neck. Card reads:

Restriction of forward flexion and extension. Pain on flexing neck to right. Good flexion to left.

Doctor asks to look at patient's eyes and fundi. Card reads:

Eye examination and fundoscopy normal.

Timing and pacing the session

It is a good idea to have a running order for the session with timings. This is especially important if multiple parallel interviews are going on in different rooms and the SPs have to move from room to room. For examinations the timetable will be strictly monitored by a dedicated timekeeper, but for teaching sessions it will be up to the facilitator(s) to keep to time. A session run in one room without break-out groups can be more flexible, and timings altered to suit the learners as long as breaks and the finishing time are adhered to: sessions that run over time may cause anxiety to some participants who have other commitments.

If the group has not worked together before, the session should start with introductions and it is also helpful for group dynamics to have an icebreaker. However there may not be time for the latter. Introductions should be kept short unless the group is small and there is plenty of time. The facilitator should then outline the session and discuss the learning objectives, exploring with the group whether these are acceptable and whether the participants wish to add to them. A generic outline for a session is shown in Box 3.3.

Example 1: an introduction to medical interviewing for first year medical students

Learning objectives

- Outline basic verbal and non-verbal communication skills.
- Discuss the importance and relevance of communication skills in clinical practice.

Box 3.3   Outline of typical session

- Welcome and introductions
- Housekeeping (location of toilets, emergency exits etc)
- Icebreaker if time
- Outline and timing of session
- Explanation of way of working (this will need to be in some detail if group has not worked with SPs before)
- Giving feedback: method to be used
- Exploration of any anxieties that group members may have/answering of questions
- Work with SPs and feedback
- Discussion of learning: have the learning objectives been met?
- Evaluation
- Finishing off, thanking the group and SPs
- De-brief with SPs (and other facilitators if present)

- Demonstrate the use of communication skills in an interview with a simulated patient.
- Demonstrate skills in feedback.

This experiential session for a year group of 100 medical students was run after an introductory lecture on communication skills and a practical session during which the students role-played patients and interviewers. They had been given advice on how to give feedback. For this session with an SP, students were in smaller groups of five, and four groups of five took part at any one time (we ran the sessions over five mornings). Therefore four teaching rooms, four facilitators and four SPs (A, B, C, D) were needed. Each SP had two roles (1, 2) and each group saw one SP twice but with a different role (*see* Table 3.1). The session could have been run with five SPs depending on the budget!

   For possible content of this type of session *see* Chapter 4.

Table 3.1   First year medical student session lasting 2.5 hours

Time	Room 1	Room 2	Room 3	Room 4
09.30–09.40: Introduction				
09.40–10.05	A1	B1	C1	D1
10.05–10.30	D1	A1	B1	C1
10.30–10.55	C1	D1	A1	B1
10.55–11.10: Break				
11.10–11.35	B2	C1	D2	A2
11.35–11.55	A2	B2	C2	D2
11.55–12.00: Finish				

Example 2: workshop on communicating risk for consultant surgeons

Postgraduate deaneries often commission workshops to enhance the communication skills of trainee and experienced doctors because of increasing litigation resulting from poor communication in the workplace. The participants requested the topic for this workshop prior to the activity. One simulated patient and one facilitator worked with eight consultants for three hours. There was also an outside speaker experienced in risk management. The format of the session was introduction, setting of learning outcomes and explanation of method of working. The speaker explored the topic of risk communication and the different ways that risk is measured. One surgeon volunteered to interact with the SP to discuss the risk of an operation. The other participants gave feedback and there was then a general discussion of risk communication, informed consent and sharing information with patients.

Example 3: workshop for GP trainers on methods of giving feedback to GP registrars and medical students on their consultation skills

This session was run for a group of 20 GP trainers for two hours with a 15-minute break in the middle. The aims were to explore different methods of teaching about the consultation and to practise giving feedback through an experiential workshop. We concentrated on two methods, each for one hour. The first method involved a volunteer medical student interviewing a simulated patient in a room separate from the main group. One GP trainer was designated as the 'tutor'. The student presented the history to the trainer who then gave feedback in whatever manner he felt appropriate. The group then gave feedback to the trainer about the teaching, following which there was a general group discussion about the method and other ways of tutoring in this format. For the second part a volunteer GP registrar interviewed an SP for 12 minutes in the presence of one of the GP trainers, as if all three were in the consulting room together, with the facilitator and other participants watching. The trainer then gave the registrar feedback with whatever method she normally used. The group and the facilitator gave feedback on the teaching process. The registrar was also asked to comment on what she found helpful when observed consulting. It is important when running such a session to keep in mind the aims. It is easy for participants to begin giving the student or the registrar feedback on their skills rather than giving feedback to the GP trainer on his/her skills. Such a session generates a lot of discussion about teaching methods, logistics and giving feedback.

Example 4: two-hour session on concordance in respect of prescribed medication for pharmacists undertaking a masters degree

The aims of this session were to discuss the concept of concordance and shared decision making between doctor and patient, and the way these relate to patient adherence to taking prescribed medication. There was one facilitator, one simulated patient and five pharmacists. The pharmacists were not used to working with an SP though they had role-played in the past. We worked through two scenarios. In the first a previously fit man was being discharged from hospital on five different tablets and was reluctant to take them all. In the second a man recently diagnosed with hypertension consulted his local pharmacist for advice about his new medication and possible side-effects. The scenarios were the basis for discussion of what happens in medical consultations, how doctors may interact with patients to make it more likely that the patient will take medication as prescribed, and the role of the pharmacist in these processes. The concept of concordance was also discussed.

This session could also be run with an interprofessional group of doctors, nurses and pharmacists.

Working with groups

The above four examples show how flexible working with SPs can be. The group size may be from one plus observer to a lecture theatre-sized audience. The bigger the group the less likely that all participants will be able to interact directly with an SP, and the aims of the session will need to be adjusted accordingly. The sessions should be interactive, and the skilled facilitator will be able to involve all participants in discussion and feedback.

In larger groups there is sometimes a problem in choosing a volunteer to interview the SP. It is great when someone does volunteer but it is possible that this person does not need as much help as someone who is quiet and would never volunteer for anything. A useful method is to give all participants on arrival a number or a raffle ticket and then draw a number from a hat or ask the SP to choose a number. This can obviously be done more than once.

The goldfish bowl technique

The sessions described above use a technique commonly called the 'goldfish bowl'. All group participants and the facilitator are in the same room watching the scenario unfold, with the interviewer and simulated patient in the spotlight (or goldfish bowl). While this is difficult for the 'performers' at the start, it allows intervention in the consultation if there are any problems, or to highlight skills parts of the interview may be re-run with ease, the interviewer may be substituted and there are few technical issues such as sound. The whole exercise is indeed very low-tech and requires no expensive equipment.

Using video

Videotaping during communication skills training is also common but obviously more expensive, and liable to go wrong, holding up proceedings. A video may be made of the interaction during a goldfish bowl session: the tape may then be played back so that the learner sees his/her body language and verbal communication in relation to the feedback being given. There is also the opportunity for the learner to keep the tape and review it privately to enhance reflection and learning. A timer on the tape helps find the relevant portion of the interview, reducing time wasting from searching through the footage.

Video may also be used to tape 'private' consultations, i.e. the interviewer and SP are in a separate room and are not watched by the group or facilitator in 'real time'. The video is reviewed by the group following this. Feedback is given in the same way as in the goldfish bowl but there is less immediacy, as the interview cannot be stopped if necessary. However different strategies may be rehearsed within the group 'live'. Being alone in a room may make the consultation feel more authentic, but probably doesn't add value to the learning experience overall.

If the facilities and technology are available, the interviewer and SP may be in a separate room being recorded and the group can watch on close-circuit television. This may help reduce the anxiety of the interviewer, the tape is available for longer-term review and there is the opportunity for the facilitator to stop the interview if appropriate. However this is a costly option.

A curriculum for communication skills: deciding on the content of sessions

SPs and scenarios may be used for skills and behaviour development beyond 'communication', though communication is a common theme in the sessions. A suggested curriculum for a typical five-year undergraduate medical programme is shown in Box 3.4. The topics will vary depending on what the students are covering in the rest of their course. It is a good idea if these skills are complementary to the knowledge and skills they are learning elsewhere. (For another suggested curriculum *see* Theo Schofield's work.[3])

Box 3.4   Possible communication learning sessions (medical students)

Year 1	Year 2
Introduction to medical interviewing	Cultural awareness
Macro- and micro-communication skills	Communicating with the deaf
Gathering information and listening	Mental health issues
The patient-centred approach	Giving a presentation
Team working	Paternalism and patient autonomy
The doctor–patient relationship	The patient's narrative
Year 3	**Year 4**
Introduction to history-taking	Interviewing children
Information sharing	Eliciting a sexual history
Working through patient encounters	Eliciting a psychiatric history
Informed consent	Compliance and concordance
Medication review	Discussing ethical issues
Year 5	
Working within a multiprofessional team	Communicating risk
Dealing with difficult situations	Working with interpreters and patient advocates
Problems with colleagues	Introduction to breaking bad news
Shared decision making	Electronic communication

Junior doctors need to practise generic skills, but they may also have specialty topics they need to cover. Skills sessions may focus on problems they bring: patients interviewed on the wards or in the community with whom they have had communication difficulties; issues relating to teamwork etc. Suggested topics are shown in Box 3.5.

Box 3.5   Scenarios for junior doctors

- The patient-centred consultation
- Shared decision making
- Breaking bad news
- Dealing with an aggressive patient or relative
- Situations involving confidentiality
- Dealing with a sick or poorly performing colleague
- Interviewing for a practice vacancy (e.g. receptionist)
- Being interviewed for a senior post
- Being appraised
- Mock clinical assessments (based on the professional examinations they will be taking)
- Working with an interpreter
- Interviewing a patient with little or no English, in the presence of a family member
- Dealing with a drug seeker
- Motivational interviewing

Senior clinicians may have specific requirements but some suggestions are given in Box 3.6.

Box 3.6   Scenarios for senior doctors/clinicians

- Carrying out an appraisal interview
- Dealing with a difficult junior: reprimanding/warning
- Dealing with a patient complaint
- Appearing in court as an expert witness
- Informed consent and risk communication
- Giving a bedside teaching session
- Giving feedback in a teaching session
- Teaching clinical skills to medical students

Evaluation

In order to gauge whether a learning session has been useful it is important to build time for evaluation into the planned activities. This may take the form of a group discussion at the end of the session or may be more formal with evaluation forms. If forms are used it is helpful if there is time built into the session for these to be filled in before participants leave in order to get as many returned as possible. This allows feedback from all participants. However short-term evaluation on the day does not allow a learner much time to reflect on what has happened and what has been learnt. Longer-term evaluation is useful to find out what knowledge and skills participants have retained from the session and to ascertain what, if anything, they have put into practice since their activity.

However, such longer-term evaluation a few weeks or even months after learning activities is extremely useful but likely to have a poor return. Medical and other students may be a captive group, but working health professionals may not see such evaluation as a priority in their busy lives. Reminders and forms by email may be the most successful method, otherwise send stamped addressed envelopes.

Some participants may be reluctant to give feedback on the day if they have not enjoyed the session or if interviewing an SP has made them feel uncomfortable. Questionnaires filled in anonymously may allow them to be more frank. But this does not facilitate discussion of their feelings. Some participants make ample use of space for free text comments, whereas others will only answer set questions or fill in Likert scales.

When deciding on what format the evaluation should take it is helpful to consider Kirkpatrick's model of evaluation. This model will help you consider what it is you are hoping to evaluate (*see* Box 3.7).[4] Remember also that questionnaires need to be read and responses counted. Any free text needs to be summarised and put into context. This is not difficult for five respondents, but for 100 or more it takes time.

Box 3.7   Different levels of evaluation (modified from Kirkpatrick)[4]

- *Learner satisfaction*: did the participants like the sessions? Were they satisfied with the content, delivery, pacing, scenarios and facilitators?
- *Learning outcomes*: did the participants learn anything? Were they satisfied with the objectives and were these met? Did they improve their skills?
- *Performance improvement*: Longer-term evaluation. Did the learners change their behaviour as a result of the activity? Are they using their new skills in their workplace?
- *Patient/health outcomes*: these are the most difficult to evaluate and are therefore often left out. With regard to communication skills, do patients notice a change in the communication behaviour of their doctor? Does this improve their healthcare?

One aspect of evaluation that is often forgotten is closing the loop: informing those who have evaluated a session what you are going to do about what they have said and/or written. If feedback was mainly positive you are probably not going to alter the session greatly for the next group. If, however, participants were unhappy with certain aspects of the sessions you should think about modifying these if possible. In particular, students become disenchanted with filling in evaluation forms, as they do not see any changes made to courses as they move up through the years. Think of ways of informing them that their feedback is being acted upon and changes made.

Summary

Planning is important, including setting objectives, choosing scenarios and working out a session timetable. Facilitators and SPs need training in the art of giving feedback. Don't forget the evaluation process.

References

1 Pendleton D, Schofield T, Tate P and Havelock P. *The Consultation: an approach to learning and teaching*. Oxford: Oxford University Press, 1984.

2 Pendleton D, Schofield T, Tate P and Havelock P. *The New Consultation. Developing doctor–patient communication*. Oxford: Oxford University Press, 2003.

3 Schofield T. A curriculum for communication in medical education. Appendix II in: Macdonald E (ed). *Difficult Conversations in Medicine*. Oxford: Oxford University Press, 2004; 209–21.

4 Kirkpatrick DI. *Evaluating Training Programs: the four levels*. San Francisco: Berrett–Koehler, 1994.

Chapter 4

Working with medical and health professional students: information gathering

This chapter explores:

- learning and teaching early communication skills
- scenarios for information gathering
- more formal history taking
- integration of content and process into consultation skills
- scenarios for eliciting medical histories.

Current trends in medical education include early patient contact. Students observe interactions between health professionals and patients from year one of their studies and are usually asked to interview patients. At this stage in their training the emphasis is on communication and information gathering rather than the more formalised and structured history taking that they learn in later years. The intelligent young people who enter medical school and the other health professions' training are already articulate, though some may be lacking in confidence. Early exposure to the patient experience and communication skills sessions should help students to talk to patients in a professional manner, while stressing the need for listening to patients' stories and developing empathy from an understanding of what it is like to be ill and/or be receiving healthcare.

There are numerous research findings that show that once students begin to 'take histories' and concentrate on disease processes they are likely to become less empathic, and indeed they often show a deterioration in their ability to communicate. They tend to interrupt patients more in order to keep their histories confined to the questions that they, the students, want answered and they begin to use medical jargon when explaining illness and procedures to patients.

Early communication skills training concentrates on the patient-centred approach, while students often become more doctor-centred as they progress through medical school. This highlights the importance of continuing to revisit and develop consultation skills throughout training, rather than confine these to the early years of the curriculum.

Communication skills training in the early years of the course

As mentioned above, health profession students come to university as good communicators though they may not be aware of the skills they are using. Early training should build on these skills. Some students feel that such training is a waste of time because of their existing proficiency; many students will have been members of school debating societies and most will have experience of community work. Thus an introduction to communication skills for health professionals should emphasise why the subject is taught, the evidence for poor communication among many trained clinicians, and the increasing litigation that often stems from lack of communication or miscommunication.

While demonstrating that there are similarities between social conversations, communications skills sessions should highlight the differences between such interactions and those between a health professional and a patient (*see* Box 4.1).

Box 4.1   Why patient interviews are different from normal social discourse

- There is often a power imbalance between clinician and patient.
- The patient is likely to be anxious and worried.
- Medical language and jargon are often indecipherable to patients.
- Clinicians ask very personal questions of someone they are meeting for the first time.
- Patients trust their clinicians and are usually very frank in their disclosures to 'a stranger'.
- Patients may not reveal their underlying ideas and concerns unless asked directly.

When asked to gather information from a patient, students often try to take a medical history even though they lack the medical knowledge and expertise to do so. Thus it is important that they are fully briefed before working with SPs as to the learning outcomes and what is expected of them. They are to elicit the patient's story and to explore the patient's ideas and concerns. Because this is the task, the patient-centred approach should be introduced and discussed prior to the experiential learning sessions.[1] Students will be able to find out about the patient's social circumstances and the effect these have on the patient's problem. The students should also be asked to explore what effects the patient's problem is having on the patient's social and family life. First and second year medical students should concentrate on the patient's experience of illness (ICEE or illness framework – *see* Box 4.2).[2] While they may be able to elicit symptoms they will be unable to any great extent to make sense of these within an illness framework, and they should be made aware of this.

Box 4.2   ICEE

The clinician explores:

- the patient's Ideas about what is wrong
- the patient's feelings (Concerns) about the illness(es)
- the impact (Effect) of the patient's problems on function/daily living
- the patient's Expectations about what should be done.

It is not within the remit of this book to go into any great depth about communication skills themselves, however Box 4.3 has a reminder of the fundamental steps in these early interviews and the language of communication of which students should be aware so that they may give and receive feedback.

Box 4.3   The language of communication

---

* Introductions including purpose of interview
* Putting the patient at ease
* Information gathering
* Listening
* Open, closed and leading questions
* Body language
* Non-verbal communication
* Encouragers
* Using pauses
* Empathy and empathic phrases
* Summarising
* Finishing off

Scenarios for information gathering

The following scenarios have been developed and delivered to first year medical students. They are all set in a general practice waiting room, as in this way the patient can 'present with' a new problem. One of the aims of the scenarios is to introduce and explain experiential learning when consulting with SPs. It is vital that the students experience a positive learning experience, as their attitude to the method will be founded here.

The whole session must run to time with the SPs delivering their roles in a consistent manner. For example the SPs should introduce themselves in role and stay in role for 95% of the session. They give feedback in role and speak to the student as the patient would, never as themselves out of role until the facilitator asks them to come out of role.

There is a tendency for experienced doctors to modify the session and do it their own way. This happens for many reasons: in part because they know what they are doing; they have misunderstood the method; they have arrived late and cannot hold all the strands of the session together; they allow the tasks to run over time having a knock-on effect with the other groups.

Some facilitators simply lack credibility because they are not used to working with small groups or with SPs and find themselves unable to orchestrate the sessions. The facilitators may allow one or more students to control the group; or one or more students to remain on the margin and not contribute to the development of the learning experience. Some facilitators feel that they need to know all the answers to a particular situation, and feel uncomfortable asking the students to work through solutions or look for answers from other related settings, for example how experienced doctors on wards might solve the problem.

Some inexperienced SPs make a bad start to their role. This may be due to their anxiety trying to remember all the detail of the role, or stage shock or lack of practice. What ever the cause of the underperformance, the SP loses student credibility. It is possible for the experienced facilitator to adapt this situation to his/her advantage. For example if the SP is playing the role of a confused patient the facilitator can attribute the worry/concern plaguing the actor to the confusion of the patient.

There are many outcomes/objectives, which may be better achieved over several consultations. Students also grasp the methodology through participation in group work not just when in the 'hot seat' of their personal consultation.

Learning objectives

- Practice of the communication skills theory they have studied
- Ability to introduce themselves to patients in a truthful, ethical and practical manner
- Experience of interviewing patients of different sex, age and social class
- Familiarity with the forms of feedback
- Comfort with the method through working in a safe learning environment
- Information-gathering skills
- Ability to explore the ideas and concerns of patients
- Appreciation of the importance of having a thread or structure forming the basis of their questions
- Understanding of the value of checking with the patient whether a point of information is correct
- Control of their nervous energy when consulting
- Ability to pace the interview
- Recognition of and ability to handle embarrassment
- Ability to work with a facilitator
- Ability to draw on the advice of their peers

Information for the facilitator

The following four scenarios are suitable for *first and second year medical students*. In the first year they introduce the SP method; are a suitable introduction for medical students' information gathering; help develop themes when talking to a patient; raise awareness of timing; facilitate early practice of communication skills; reduce anxiety when talking to patients; help students to learn to give and receive constructive feedback.

In the second year, students can concentrate on building patient relationships; allowing the patient to speak, using open questions; summarising the interview; closing the interview; acknowledging the patient's idea of his/her illness; finding out what is worrying the patient; what symptoms can be explained to the patient; avoidance of giving false reassurance; practising empathy statements; empathising with patients.

Scenarios for junior medical students

The scenarios are given with **ICEE** for ease of use and to highlight the importance of this for junior students.

Scenario 1: mature male

> **Simulated patient**
> 'Frank Thompson age 40–50 years. I work in human resources in a large department store in the centre of town.'
>
> **Location**
> 'I am waiting in a general practice surgery, I have an appointment to see the GP and the student must request an interview with me before I go in to see the doctor.'
>
> **Medical records**
> 'I take no other medication apart from the odd paracetamol. In the past I had my appendix out aged 18.'

Activity and information for the SP

You would be dressed smart casual. You look tired and irritable. You are usually a good communicator of feelings if asked about them; you have no preconceived ideas or issues about talking to a medical student.

To build up a good character you should talk to a friend or colleague who has had acid indigestion. Good questions to ask about are: the strength of pain your indigestion has caused you; the position and spread of the pain; how much does the pain disturb your sleep; what worries does the indigestion cause you, your wife, your family; has it caused problems at work directly; whether you lack the ability to concentrate on your job because you did not sleep normally; if food in the staff restaurant causes or inflames your problem; because of the problem have you changed your personality, for example are you less humorous/easy going than normal?

> **Background information**
> 'I have always had to watch what I eat as I suffer with indigestion after rich and spicy foods. Usually any indigestion settles with medicine I buy from the pharmacy (Asilone or Gaviscon). Over the last month I have been getting more pain that is worse than usual and it sometimes wakes me at night. I get the pain most days now and it doesn't seem to matter what I eat. The pain is just below my ribs in the centre, and sometimes I also get an acid taste in my mouth.'
>
> **Expectations**
> 'I would like the doctor to give me something to stop the pain and I would be happy with this suggestion.
>
> On a deeper level I am *concerned* as I think I may have an ulcer and I might like some tests to make sure I do not. I have an *idea* that I have lost weight because something is seriously wrong. I have lost a few kilos – people with cancer lose weight as one of their symptoms; although I expect to talk about this I would not raise these concerns first, nor until I felt comfortable with the interviewer.'
>
> **Summary**
> - 'I get the pain at night; it keeps me awake for 1–2 hours.
> - I am married and everything is fine at home.
> - My wife Anne is concerned about the pain and has been repeatedly telling me to go to the doctor's.
> - My bowels are OK.

Continued

> - I take no other medication apart from the odd paracetamol for infrequent headaches.
> - When I was 18 I had my appendix out.'

Points for discussion

There should be some discussion concerning what students learn from this scenario and what can go wrong, e.g. wrong introduction, talking over the patient, poor structure to questions; not uncovering the fear of cancer.

Scenario 2: mature female

> **Simulated patient**
> 'Cathy Townsend, aged 50+ years. I work as a tourist information officer in a busy town centre office.'
>
> **Location**
> 'I am waiting in a GP surgery and the student requests an interview.'
>
> **Medical records**
> 'I have had 3 children and an inguinal hernia (groin) repair. I have high blood pressure controlled by lisinopril, this was diagnosed five years ago and is usually well controlled.'

Activity and information for the SP

Talk to a colleague who has suffered some kind of anxiety attack brought on by the fear of doing an ordinary action leading to a loss of confidence, possibly where good counselling has helped the person regain confidence instead of medication. Be familiar with recent newsworthy events that may concern travellers.

> **Background information**
> 'I am planning a trip overseas to see my son and his family who live in Bahrain. I am quite anxious about this due to my *ideas* about the possibility of terrorist activity in the Middle East recently. The anxiety has kept me awake at night thinking about the flight. I am also *concerned* about the possibility of blood clots in the leg on such a long flight . . . they can kill you can't they? I have high blood pressure and take treatment for this. I do not smoke. Things are getting so bad now that I almost feel as if I can't make the trip, surely my blood pressure will go up. I will be travelling on my own as my husband died of a heart attack three years ago. I still miss him. My friend thinks there may be something I could take to help the anxiety. I *expect* to get some kind of tranquilliser for the flight.
>
> - I haven't seen my son for three years.
> - I have a new grandchild age 1. I am longing to see her.'

Points for discussion

How much information may a student give to a patient? Does the student give the patient false reassurance of the unlikelihood of a terrorist attack? Should the student give good advice about leg movement to improve circulation, drinking plenty of fluids on the trip and avoiding alcohol?

Scenario 3: young male

Simulated patient
'I am Steven Johnson age mid-20s; I have been working as a teacher in a large 11–16 age range school. I am open, happy, and easy to talk to.'

Location
'I am waiting in a GP surgery and the student requests an interview.'

Medical records
'Mild asthma as a child but I no longer take medication for this.'

Background information
'I am on holiday here from Australia where I work as a teacher. I have taken six months off to travel round the world before settling back into a full-time job. I have been to India and Thailand, and am now spending 10 days in England. I have been travelling for the last four months.

I have felt tired for the last two weeks and I am getting a bit breathless when I exercise. I used to run most mornings for about 8 km. Now I find it difficult to get out of bed. I do not have diarrhoea nor a cough. I am worried by my lack of fitness; all sorts of *concerns* are going through my head.'

Concerns
'Malaria; I have been taking anti-malaria tablets but I often forget them. So I think my problem is connected to the tablets: either taking them (side-effects) or not (getting malaria) may be a cause of the problem. It could even be some other virus; I have heard there are some odd ones in India.

I have had sex with a couple of girls on my travels but I used condoms. Could I have caught something?

What if I have to go home early; if I'm sick here will my insurance cover it?'

Ideas about problem
'This is something to do with travelling but I am not sure how serious it is. If only I could *expect* some reassurance and thorough physical examination, and some blood tests to test for infection. Do I need an HIV test?'

Scenario 4: young female

Simulated patient
'I am Sally Barlow aged 19, a biology student at the local university. I started the course this year.'

Location
'I am waiting in a GP surgery and a student requests an interview. I am a little shocked that someone my own age wants to interview me about personal issues.'

Medical records
'I have had no medical problems in the past.'

Continued

Background information

'My *idea* about my problem is that I am feeling homesick and I miss my boyfriend Jed, who is in London (he is 25 and works for a publishing company). I have been going out with him for two years. I am not sure I like the course and I really am *concerned* about staying on the course. I am living in halls of residence and it is noisy at night-time. I feel a bit left out socially as all the other students I have met so far are single and most of the girls seem to be looking for partners. Many students don't seem to worry much about one-night stands. I don't want to be unfaithful to Jed, but I do wonder what he is getting up to in the big city without me.

I do not drink too much alcohol or take any drugs.

I used to ride my bike to museums and to see friends but I do not feel motivated to here. It is cold and windy here. I am not eating much and I have gone off my food. I have missed a few early lectures as well because I find it hard to get up in the morning. I am not sleeping very well because of the noise. I cannot drop off to sleep and often get woken up by the noise in the early hours when other students come back to their rooms. My main *reason* for coming to the doctor is to get a certificate because I missed some lectures and a test yesterday. I do not really want to talk to the doctor. I will just say that I feel a bit run down. I may even ask for sleeping tablets, I do not want any other pills but I will accept them if any are offered.

I *expect* to get a certificate of illness to excuse my absence from lectures but I would really like to discuss my problem at an emotional level. If I am asked more in a gentle and sympathetic way I will say why I am tired and I will explain about not sleeping. Also Jed was supposed to be coming to stay in the lecture break next week, but he has asked me to go back home, as he is too busy to make it.

I have not told Jed or my parents how low I am feeling.'

Points for discussion

Scenarios relating to patients about the same age as the medical students may contain some issues that the medical students themselves are working through, particularly homesickness, boyfriend/girlfriend problems etc. The group can discuss whether having similar problems to patients helps with empathy. Does it make the consultation too personal? Does the age of a patient affect how the students feel and communicate?

More formal 'history taking'

Medical students tend to learn the art of history taking in year two or even three of an undergraduate course, and year two of a graduate course. By this time they should have a good grounding in communication skills and information gathering. One way of introducing the new skills they need in relation to the medical history is to explore with the students the tasks of the doctor–patient interaction, i.e. those areas that should be discussed with the patient. Such tasks may be referred to as the content of the interaction or consultation. Communication skills are the means by which the doctor or student achieves the tasks: the process. Content and process have all too often been treated as separate entities. Together the tasks of the consultation and the communication skills needed may be referred to as consultation skills. Such integration thus marries the task-orientated consultation with the patient-centred behavioural approach, as outlined in the Calgary–Cambridge model.[3]

Whereas the early communication skills scenarios concentrate on students gathering information about a patient's problems and the effects of these (ICEE), history taking aims to gather information about a patient's symptoms in order for the doctor/student to formulate a differential diagnosis and/or problem list. Students should be encouraged to think about the diagnostic process and the ways in which a diagnosis is made: the combination of the hypothetical–deductive model and pattern recognition. Tutors should also stress that patients do not always consult for a diagnosis, especially in primary care settings where students often begin to practise their history taking.

When introducing the medical history it is interesting to discuss the use of language and the message this conveys about the doctor–patient relationship: *take* a history. Discuss alternatives. What words could be used for this process? We prefer *elicit* a history, but the phrase '*building* a history' has also been used.[4] The concept of the patient's narrative is also helpful. As defined by Greenhalgh and Hurwitz, academic GPs in London, 'the narrative context of illness provides a framework for approaching a patient's problem holistically, as well as revealing potential diagnostic and therapeutic options'.[5]

Box 4.4   The traditional medical history

- The presenting complaint
- History of the present illness
- Previous history of illness
- Menstrual history
- Treatment history
- Family history
- Social history
- Personal history
- Psychiatric history
- (Systems review)

The familiar structure of the traditional medical history is given in Box 4.4. As taught by some clinicians and practised by many students, the social history consists merely of where the patient lives, with whom and in what sort of accommodation. The personal history relates to smoking, alcohol and drug use. Students need to be reminded of the patient-centred approach and ICEE, and helped to integrate this with the formal history. The idea of the psychosocial history is also important, in much more depth where relevant than the bare social and personal histories. In spite of its limitations students usually find the formalised structure helpful, with the tasks of the consultation clearly delineated. More experienced students should be able to work through both the patient's and their own agendas while being mindful of the desired outcome of the consultation for both participants. Box 4.5 is useful as a handout to draw attention to what patients have been found to want from consultations.[6]

Before students do begin to elicit histories from patients in general practice and in hospital, the differences between the types of histories expected from the patients' clinicians should be discussed, as well as what is appropriate and relevant if a patient is very sick in contrast to one who is fairly well or has a non-life-threatening condition. However to avoid confusion, students need to be reminded that in almost all cases a patient-centred approach and exploration of a patient's anxieties is good practice.

Box 4.5   What patients want from consultations

- Exploration of the main reason for consultation
- Integrated understanding of patient's world (whole person, emotional needs, life issues)
- Common ground as to the nature of the problem
- Mutual agreement on management
- Enhancement of health promotion and disease prevention
- Enhancement of the doctor–patient relationship

Scenarios for eliciting histories

The following two scenarios are written with the aim of helping medical students realise the importance of the psychosocial history and the patient-centred approach in the diagnosis of a patient's presenting complaint. Suggestions for running the sessions are given after the scenarios.

Patient presenting to the out-of-hours GP clinic with previous chest pain

Simulated patient
'I am Paul Barker, a 52-year-old gardener with my own landscaping business.'

Three weeks ago I had a bout of chest pain in the morning while I was working on a garden . . . digging etc. The pain was in the centre of my chest and didn't go anywhere else. I thought it was likely to be indigestion as I had had a big meal the night before as it was my wedding anniversary. I stopped work for about 20 minutes and had a cup of tea; the pain settled.

About one week ago I had a similar episode while working. The pain again was in the centre of my chest. I had to stop. I felt a bit sweaty. The pain lasted about 15 minutes and then I was able to carry on working, though didn't do anything too much. I thought it could still be indigestion. I took a Rennie (indigestion pill) and thought that must have helped.

Today I had similar pain but also some pain in my left shoulder. I stopped and sat down in the garden. The owner saw me and was worried. She was going to call an ambulance but the pain stopped after about 15 minutes. I promised to see a doctor. I felt sweaty again and dizzy. I told my wife when I got home. She insisted I see a doctor straight away so now here I am at the out-of-hours GP clinic.'

Past medical history
'I am usually fit and well. I have occasional indigestion, and take Rennies about once every few months. I have no other symptoms with this. I've had it for years. Appendicectomy age 18. I had my blood pressure checked at the pharmacy about one year ago and was told it was normal.

I smoked between the ages of 16 and 50, about five to ten per day. Nothing since then. I rarely drink except on special occasions.

I live with my wife. She has a heart valve problem and is on lots of medication. We have no children. I take no other drugs.'

Continued

Ideas and concerns
'I hope this is indigestion but the third episode has made me wonder about my heart. If I have a heart problem, how will that affect my business? I need to be active at work. I employ two young lads but they do need supervision. I have spent a lot of time building up my business and don't want to lose custom.'

Patient presenting in general practice with a cough

Simulated patient
'I am Michael Porter, a 48-year-old bar manager.'
   I have had a cough for three weeks. I want more antibiotics. I had some antibiotics a week ago from another doctor here and they helped a bit. I am sure another course will clear my chest.
   I have had a morning cough for years. I cough up a bit of phlegm (white or dirty) then I am OK for the rest of the day. This new cough occurs at any time. Most times I don't cough up anything but yesterday I coughed up a few streaks of blood. My daughter saw this and told me to see a doctor again. I am coughing at night and this keeps me awake. I need my sleep as I work long hours. I have probably lost a few kilos in the last few weeks.'

Past medical history
'I usually get a chest infection about once a year that clears quickly. I had a broken arm about 16 years ago. I smoke 30 a day plus marijuana and take cocaine occasionally. I drink four pints of lager a night during work and then a few tots of whisky to help me sleep.
   My wife left me two months ago; she says because of my drinking but I think she has another bloke. My daughter (20) helps in the bar but she is about to move to London with her boyfriend. I have a son age 30 from a previous relationship, but I never see him.'

Ideas
'I just want things clearing up. I know I drink too much, but what the hell. I tried to give up about 10 years ago but was not successful and the amount has gradually increased since then. There is nothing wrong with smoking the odd joint either and I'm certainly not addicted to cocaine.'

Concerns
'I suppose the cough could be due to something more serious. But I haven't got time to have tests as I need to run the bar or I'll lose it and my flat (above it).'

Notes for facilitators

Chest pain and cough are two common presenting complaints. They may be due to easily resolved conditions or there may be more sinister underlying causes in these cases. The students need to be able to elicit the history to decide on a differential diagnosis, but also to listen to the patient's story in terms of their life stresses and concerns, as these have a bearing on what will happen next. Both men are concerned about the possible effects of their condition on their jobs. Paul will be amenable to any suggestions with regard to investigations, as he wants to get back his good health and carry on with his business. Michael has several problems that need exploring and tackling, including his drinking and smoking. The students may not probe enough to discover the extent of Michael's drinking, or find out about his illicit drug use. Even though the scenarios are written to help students practise eliciting histories, the students can also be asked to think about what should happen next.

Ways of working through the scenarios

The aim of the learning experience is to help students integrate history taking with communication skills and the patient-centred approach. They may have learnt the latter a few years ago, while they have been taught the more formal history-taking process recently.

Method 1

This is suitable for groups of up to 12 students. The students sit in a circle. One student 'volunteers' to start. This student invites the SP to enter the room and sit down in the empty chair next to the student. The student introduces him/herself and begins the interview. When he/she cannot think of what to ask next, or at an appropriate point, the student passes on the role of interviewer to the student sitting next to him. This carries on until no-one can think of any more questions to ask. At this point the facilitator asks the next student to present the history as elicited so far and makes notes on a flip chart. The facilitator then asks from the data gathered so far what the students think is the differential diagnosis. Why do they think this? What further questions do they need to ask to narrow down the list? If there are any more questions, a student asks the SP. The facilitator asks the group what they think are the patient's ideas and concerns. If these have not been elicited during the interview, a student now explores them with the patient.

At the end of this process the students are asked to formulate a problem list for the patient and to check that this is accurate with the SP. Paul's problem list will include:

- chest pain: cause?
- physically active job
- concerns about his business if he has a heart condition.

Paul will agree with all these.
Michael's will include:

- cough: cause?
- heavy smoker
- heavy drinker
- illicit drug user
- unstable lifestyle due to marriage breakdown
- daughter about to leave
- possible problems with job and accommodation if there is a serious health problem.

Michael may not agree that all these are a problem. This can be discussed.

The students are then asked to comment on their communication skills. What did they do well? What could be done differently to help the story unfold? How did they feel about asking about drinking and illicit drugs? The SP is then asked to comment on the types of questions asked. What felt comfortable? What didn't? Is there any further information the students should have?

At the end of each scenario, the facilitator could ask the students what should be done next in terms of investigations. At this stage the students may not have much knowledge about this, but they will be interested in knowing what should happen next.

The facilitator points out the integration of the history taking with the patient-centred approach: this is vital to understand the patient's story and their reaction to the possible diagnosis and management plan.

Method 2

This works better with a smaller group of students. A student interviews the SP in a separate room and this is videotaped. If there is close circuit television, the group watches the interaction.[7] If not, the tape is watched after the interview with the SP in role (more time consuming). One of the watching students is asked to present the history. If more questions need to be asked, one of the group asks the SP. The session then carries on as with method 1. This method is more realistic in terms of the interview process, but means that it is unlikely, depending on the size of the group, that all the students will have a chance to interview the patient.

Summary

Experiential learning is important for students in their early years of learning to communicate and elicit histories. They need to be reminded about the patient-centred approach and receive constructive and timely feedback.

References

1   Levenstein JH, McCracken EC, McWhinney IR *et al*. The patient-centred clinical method. 1. A model for the doctor–patient interaction in family medicine. *Fam Pract*. 1986; **3**: 24–30.
2   Stewart M and Roter D. *Communicating with Medical Patients*. Newbury: Sage Publications, 1989.
3   Kurtz S, Silverman J, Benson J and Draper J. Marrying content and process in clinical method teaching: enhancing the Calgary–Cambridge guides. *Acad Med*. 2003; **78**: 802–9.
4   Haidet P and Paterniti DA. 'Building' a history rather than 'taking' one: a perspective on information sharing during the medical interview. *Arch Int Med*. 2003; **163**: 1134–40.
5   Greenhalgh T and Hurwitz B. Why study narrative? In: Greenhalgh T and Hurwitz B (eds). *Narrative Based Medicine*. London: BMJ Books, 1998, pp 3–29.
6   Stewart M. Towards a global definition of patient centred care. *BMJ*. 2001; **322**: 444–5.
7   Thistlethwaite JE. Integrating communication skills and history-taking. *Med Teach*. 1999; **21**: 83–4.

Chapter 5

Information sharing and shared decision making

This chapter explores:

- background research relating to information sharing
- information needs of patients
- shared decision making and scenarios
- adherence, compliance and concordance
- wants and needs of patients.

Health professionals spend a great deal of their time giving information and advice to patients. Patients may specifically ask for information on a given topic when they consult, or the information and advice may be part of the management plan following diagnosis.

The skill for a trainee to learn is the ability to translate medical terminology (or jargon) into language that the patient may understand. What words and terms are used will depend on the prior knowledge of the patient, which may be related to their occupation, educational attainment, age and/or cultural background. Explanation may need to be given about investigations, how procedures are performed, how a particular disease or condition may affect the patient, long-term effects of the condition or treatment, what treatment options are available, their side-effects and so on.

In terms of management the model of patient partnership and shared decision making requires skill building. Trainees need to be aware that most patients no longer want to be told what to do, and experienced clinicians may need to move away from a paternalistic framework into a more patient-centred approach.

Learning objectives for information-sharing sessions

- Exploration and understanding of the information needs of patients
- Assessment of prior knowledge of patients
- Ability to give medical information in a clear and understandable manner
- Knowledge of how to check patient understanding
- Competencies for shared decision making
- Discussion of rationale behind information sharing and shared decision making (improved patient adherence, likelihood of concordance in consultation)

Background information from the literature

This information may be covered in an introductory session or could be discussed after the experiential learning session. The facilitator may be able to help the students define what patients want to know and what type of information is necessary. The bullet points in Box 5.1 should be useful for students and could be given out as handouts.

Scenarios for information sharing and shared decision making

Information sharing: basic explanation

For:

Junior health professional and medical students who are beginning to learn about common medical conditions but do not have knowledge of medication or treatment options as yet. Students may be asked to explain in lay person's terms to an SP the basic science and underlying pathology of common conditions: the 'understanding of what is wrong' as listed in Box 5.1. Students who have some experience of common investigative procedures may also be asked to explain these: the processes and likely outcomes of possible tests. Suitable topics include: hypertension, type 2 diabetes, what exactly is a heart attack, what happens at endoscopy (gastroscopy or sigmoidoscopy), the exercise electrocardiogram (ECG). For these scenarios students can be asked to 'play the role' of a newly qualified professional.

Patient

William Morris, age mid-50s. Previously fit and well. Returning to see his GP after blood pressure readings over several weeks.

Location

General practice. The student may be asked to be a pre-registration house officer (intern) in general practice. The doctor has not seen this patient before: he has been consulting with the practice nurse who has advised him now to see the doctor.

Medical records (to be given to interviewer)

William Morris. Came for holiday vaccinations for travel to Egypt. Seen by practice nurse. Routine BP [blood pressure] measurement: 168/96 mmHg. Advised to return for check in one week. Has had three checks now over three months (been to Egypt in this time, no problems). Average BP reading 172/98 mmHg. Stopped smoking five years ago (was 20/day); 14 units alcohol per week (wine). PMH (past medical history): vasectomy age 36.

FH (family history): father died aged 66, MI (myocardial infarction); mother died age 84, bronchopneumonia.

Examination

Weight 85 kg, body mass index (BMI) 27, urinalysis negative, ECG NAD. Blood tests all within the normal range apart from total cholesterol 6.2 mmol/l. Advised to see GP to discuss high blood pressure.

Instructions to the interviewer

William Morris age mid-50s is coming to see you. He has been seeing the practice nurse. See medical records. He has not seen you before. He is coming to see you on the advice of the nurse to discuss his results and for management of his high blood pressure. Please advise the patient.

Scenario for the SP

'I am William Morris. I am an accountant. I came to have holiday vaccinations and the nurse checked my blood pressure. She told me it was slightly raised. I have had it checked twice since then and it has been up. I have had some blood tests and an ECG. The nurse advised me to see my GP for the results and further management. I have not seen this doctor before as I rarely come to the doctor's. I have always thought myself to be fit for my age especially since giving up smoking five years ago. I don't do much exercise apart from a few walks at the weekends, about three miles. But I feel I eat a fairly healthy diet (no fried food and fast food rarely) though my weight has crept up over the last few years. I was surprised to hear I had raised blood pressure. I enjoy my work, have a good home life and am not particularly stressed.'

Ideas
'I don't know much about raised blood pressure, though I think it can cause strokes. I know high cholesterol is bad for you so I will be interested to know what mine is like, though I don't know anything about the figures.'

Concerns
'I feel well so I'm not too worried. My father died of a heart attack but he was a heavy smoker. I'm not sure if high blood pressure is related to heart attacks.'

Expectations
'I expect the doctor to tell me more about my blood pressure and suggest some ways to bring it down. Though I know people take tablets for blood pressure I would hope I would not need to.'

SP training

To increase authenticity of this scenario, SPs could be asked for their ideas and concerns relating to the diagnosis of high blood pressure (hypertension). It is possible that of a group of SPs in their 50s one or two may be on treatment. The role could be adapted to include these feelings and responses to diagnosis. In a teaching session the absolute details of the role are not important to achieve the outcome of being able to explain a medical condition, its possible sequelae and management options taking into account the patient's perspective. SPs should discuss whether William would ask the doctor to explain words he did not understand or would let them go (and advise the learner during feedback that the explanation was not fully understood).

Notes for facilitators

Feedback to students from all sources should include advice about checking the patient's prior knowledge, use of jargon, clear explanation of both hypertension and the slightly raised cholesterol and advice about lifestyle modification. At this consultation lifestyle modification (increased exercise, attention to diet) would be the main advice, especially as the patient does not want medication. Patient feedback is especially important: was the level and content of the explanation appropriate?

Medical students begin to use jargon fairly early on in their course and should be made aware of this through feedback from the SP either during the consultation or in the formal feedback process. There may be a tendency for the learner to do most of the talking in this consultation and this is another area to cover in feedback: how might this be avoided when giving explanations and advice? It is important to establish rapport with William, as he will need regular follow-up over the years.

Shared decision making: prescribing medication

This scenario follows on from the one above, though it could be adapted to be a new consultation. This may follow a theoretical discussion about shared decision making (SDM) or, following the scenario, the principles of SDM could be worked out by the learning group on the basis of the experience of this consultation and its outcomes.

For:

Medical students with clinical experience and knowledge of simple prescribing, GP registrars, medical registrars.

Location

GP surgery.

Patient

William Morris, three months after previous consultation.

Medical records

As above. Plus: Last consultation – discussed diagnosis and risk of hypertension. Advised regular exercise, diet and weight loss. Discussed slightly raised cholesterol. Diet sheets given. Review 3 months for BP check. Today: nurse has checked BP = 170/98 mmHg, weight 83 kg, BMI 27.

Instructions to the interviewer

William Morris is returning to see you after three months to have his blood pressure checked. Last time he saw the GP registrar who has since left the practice. His blood pressure is still raised.

Scenario for the SP

'I have tried to increase the amount of exercise I do, I still walk at the weekends, sometimes three miles, sometimes five miles. I have found it difficult to exercise during the week. I did join a gym for a month's trial but didn't like the atmosphere and found the treadmill boring. I only went three times. I am happy that I have lost a few kilos (but thought it was more!) but don't really see how I can eat less than I do. I think that now the doctor will suggest medication as I have read some things about blood pressure on the internet. I realise there are quite a few different types of tablets available. I am still not keen on tablets but will try them if the doctor gives me a good reason to do so. I expect the doctor to discuss the various side-effects and benefits of the different drugs.'

Notes for facilitators

The ideal here is for the learner to use a shared decision-making framework to involve the patient in the decision to take medication. The learner may discuss risk and use a risk calculator, or be more direct and discuss the merits of drug therapy. William wishes to be informed. He expects some say in the decision but is prepared to try tablets if he is informed about possible side-effects.

Box 5.2 shows the information that patients want about prescribed medication. Has the learner included these points?

Box 5.2   Essential information about drugs[2]

- Side-effects
- What it does and what it's for
- Dos and don'ts
- How to take it

The framework for shared decision making for discussion is in Box 5.3.

Box 5.3   Characteristics of shared decision making[3]

- Both the patient and the doctor are involved
- Both parties share information
- Both parties take steps to build a consensus about the preferred treatment
- Doctor and patient reach an agreement on the treatment to implement

---

The choice of antihypertensive medication is not crucial in this scenario, however the 'doctor' should be able to discuss the merits and side-effects of the particular drug chosen. The discussion should not be sidetracked into considering the evidence for and against different drugs as first-line treatment, though the facilitator may wish to raise the question as to whether the shared decision is solely about whether William should take medication or also includes his choice of drug.

In role the SP may give feedback on how he feels about being given a choice of medication or whether, once he has decided to take a drug, he is happy for the doctor to decide on the best drug.

Issues relating to adherence

For:

Senior medical students, pre-registration pharmacists, medical and GP registrars. The outcomes for the learner are an understanding of why patients do not always take their medication as prescribed. The debriefing session could lead into a discussion of the concepts of compliance, adherence and concordance. The importance of shared decision making for optimum medicine taking should be highlighted.

Patient

William Morris as above.

Location

A GP surgery or outpatient department. If the same group as the previous scenario are working through this case, the interviewer may assume he/she has seen the patient before and prescribed the tablets.

Scenario for the SP

'Three months ago I was prescribed the beta-blocker bisoprolol for my high blood pressure, hypertension as the doctor called it. I returned to see my doctor after one month and my BP was lower. I felt really pleased. However in the last few weeks I have been feeling more tired than usual. My sleep is being interrupted by vivid dreams that are approaching nightmares in quality. I am sure this must be due to the tablets and I stopped taking them three weeks ago, and I have to admit I now feel better. I don't really want to tell the doctor I have stopped taking the tablets as he/she had told me they were necessary. I want to discuss all this with the doctor and I will say I have stopped taking them if I am asked directly about taking the medication. If the doctor asks about side-effects I will say I have been feeling tired.'

Instructions for the doctor

William Morris is returning for a follow-up appointment. He was diagnosed with hypertension six months ago. Initially he tried lifestyle changes to reduce his blood pressure, but this did not work satisfactorily. Therefore three months ago you started him on bisoprolol and he seemed to be happy with this outcome. Two months ago his blood pressure was lower at 138/88 mmHg. Today his blood pressure is 156/98 mmHg.

Notes for facilitators

This scenario checks whether the doctor considers non-adherence as a reason for the rise in blood pressure after a previously satisfactory reading. The doctor may assume that an increase in medication or the addition of another drug is required. Or the plan may be for

William to carry on 'taking the pills' and to return for a further measurement in another month. William may also have other side-effects of the treatment, in particular impotence. This side-effect is rarely asked about and is a good opportunity for learners to practise eliciting a sexual history.

The decision whether to prescribe antibiotics

Shared decision making is more likely to happen when there are several treatment options each of which has advantages and disadvantages. One of the topics that is often raised when discussing patient involvement in the decision-making process is antibiotic prescribing. The pressure to reduce the prescribing of antibiotics for self-limiting and viral illnesses is well known. Many patients are also less likely to want antibiotics and often are seeking reassurance rather than medication. However doctors may believe, rightly or wrongly, that a patient is hoping for antibiotics. This scenario aims to facilitate a discussion of the decision-making processes resulting from a consultation in which antibiotics may or may not be prescribed. A positive outcome will be both the doctor and the patient ending the consultation feeling satisfied with what has happened. Note: there is no 'right' or 'wrong' way of conducting the interview; the success does not lie in whether antibiotics are prescribed or not.

For:

Senior medical students, GP registrars, GPs, nurse practitioners.

Location

General practice surgery.

Scenario for the SP (male or female)

'I am in my 20s. I have had a terrible sore throat for two days and am finding it increasingly difficult to swallow. I have had sore throats in the past. In my teens I used to get antibiotics several times a year for tonsillitis. Since then I have perhaps had a sore throat once a year. I last visited the GP about nine months ago with a bad throat and cold and the doctor advised me that this was a viral infection. I was happy with this explanation and in fact the symptoms only lasted a few days. However this throat is the worst I can remember since I was at school. I feel hot and my glands feel swollen. I have been having paracetamol but this does not seem to help. I cannot sleep. I am an accounts clerk and am due to go away at the weekend for a hen/stag party. I would like antibiotics as I feel so bad. I intend to ask for them if the doctor does not offer to prescribe. (If female: I am on the combined contraceptive pill.) I have no other past medical history of note. I smoke socially about five cigarettes in an evening three times a week. I drink several glasses of wine/lagers at weekends when out with friends. I take no recreational drugs.'

Instructions for the doctor

AB age 20+. 9/12 ago: viral infection: sore throat and runny nose. Throat red, ears and chest clear. Advised paracetamol. (If female: 6/12 ago: repeat prescription Microgynon 30: no problems, BP 110/60 mmHg, smokes 5–10/week). 5 years ago: tonsillitis with exudates. Treatment: 10-day course of penicillin V.

Examination of the patient

Enlarged tonsils with crypts seen. No exudate. Cervical glands swollen. Right TM (tympanic membrane): pink, left TM: NAD. Chest clear.

Notes for facilitators

Possible outcomes of this consultation are:

1 No prescription. The patient is told they have a viral infection and will get better on their own. There is no discussion and the patient is not happy. They may try to get a second opinion.
2 No prescription. The doctor discusses treatment decision with the patient. The patient is happy.
3 The doctor discusses pros and cons of antibiotic prescribing and asks for the patient's opinion. The patient wishes to have a prescription, therefore one is given.
4 As 3, but the doctor advised patient to wait 24–48 hours to see if symptoms resolve before getting the medication.
5 There may also be a discussion of the possibility of glandular fever. However a treatment decision should be made on this occasion.

This can lead onto a discussion about the wants and needs of patients. The SP should be involved in this and talk about expectations and the best way (in his/her opinion) for the doctor to handle the situation.

Explanation of test results

For:

Senior medical students, gynaecology registrars, GP registrars, practice nurses, sexual health nurses.

Scenario for the SP

'I am Sarah; I am 26 years old and a waitress. I have been on the oral contraceptive pill Microgynon for 10 years. I have been with my current boyfriend for six months. We do not use condoms. Prior to this I have had about six sexual partners. Sometimes I used condoms, sometimes I didn't: it depended on whether my partner wanted to, or whether I was drunk. I tested positive for Chlamydia one year ago and was treated with a one-off dose of an antibiotic. Two weeks ago I had my second cervical smear. I had my first when I was 22. I didn't hear anything about it so I assume it was OK. The doctor who treated my Chlamydia said I should have another but I didn't get round to it until I needed some more pills. The nurse took my smear. I got a letter saying it has a slight abnormality and I have to come and talk to someone about the result. I am a bit worried. I wonder if I have another infection or even if I have cancer, though I think that they pick that up early on a smear and treat it so it shouldn't be too bad. I wish I hadn't left it so long to have the smear. I want to know the answers to the following questions, but will only be able to ask if the doctor/nurse seems OK and I don't think they are judging me because of my sexual habits:

- are there any signs of another sexually transmitted infection?
- do I have cancer?

Continued

- if there is something really bad with this smear could it have been missed on the first one?
- is it because I am late with this one?
- is it because I don't use condoms?
- is it my boyfriend's fault?
- is it related to the previous infection?
- will it affect me having children? (I will want children eventually.)'

Information for the clinician: medical notes

Sarah age 26 years. Seen 2 weeks ago. Repeat prescription for Microgynon. BP 110/70 mmHg. Smokes 10/day. Advised to stop. Due smear. About 4 years since last one. 1 year ago, treated for Chlamydia (urine test). LMP (last menstrual period): 2 weeks ago. O/E (examination): cervical ectopy. No discharge seen. Smear taken.

Cervical smear result: satisfactory smear. Endocervical cells present. CIN 1 with HPV (human papillomavirus). Advised repeat smear in 6 months.

Extra notes for the SP

If you do not think that the explanation of the smear result is clear for you, you may ask to see a specialist for further tests rather than wait 6 months. If the doctor uses the terms pre-cancer or wart virus you want to know exactly what these mean. Do you have genital warts? Should you have these treated? What about your boyfriend? Will he have warts that need treating? Does he need to see a doctor?

Notes for facilitators

This is a very common scenario and tests the clinician's ability to share medical information in a way that the patient will understand. The attitudes of the group to behaviour like Sarah's may also be discussed. What is the role of the clinician in health promotion in this case? Again in this case there are issues relating to Sarah's wants and needs. If she continues to feel anxious after discussion of her results, she may insist on seeing a gynaecologist, though this is not necessary according to the recommendation of the cytologist.

Summary

Information sharing and shared decision making are important skills for health professionals. Working through cases with SPs helps professionals understand the need to use accessible language and check understanding.

References

1 Coulter A, Entwistle V and Gilbert D. Sharing decisions with patients: is the information good enough? *BMJ*. 1999; **318**: 318–22.

2 Dickinson D and Raynor DKT. Ask the patients – they may want to know more than you think. *BMJ*. 2003; **327**: 861.

3 Charles C, Gafni A and Whelan T. Shared decision-making in the medical encounter: what does it mean? (or it takes two to tango). *Soc Sci Med*. 1997; **44**: 681–92.

Chapter 6

Risk communication and informed consent

This chapter explores:

- the concept of risk communication and the language of risk
- scenarios relating to risk communication
- informed consent.

We all indulge in risky behaviour and weigh up the benefits and possible bad effects in various ways, depending on personality and experience. Health professionals have to convey the notion of risk in such a way that patients may understand the choices they face. Different people will react in different ways to risk data, thus communication needs to be individually tailored to take into account how patients handle figures and what they are prepared to gain or lose. Only if a patient fully understands the risks he or she faces can they truly give informed consent. In the past, the paternalistic doctor often gave minimal information about risk in order to shield the patient from worry. This behaviour is no longer acceptable as patients have a legal as well as a moral right to understand their illness and the possible benefits or adverse risks of treatment options.

Learning objectives for risk communication

- Understanding the language of risk
- Differentiation between absolute, relative risk and number needed to treat
- Ability to transfer technical information to a patient relating to treatment options, risks and their probable benefits in an unbiased, clear and simple way
- Ability to help a patient conceptualise the weighing process of risks versus benefits and ensuring that preferences are based on fact and not misconception

Background to the language of risk

Risk means the possibility of suffering harm or loss. In the context of medicine patients need to be informed of the risk due to their illness or condition, the risk of treatment and the risk of non-treatment. There may also be the potential of harm to others e.g. a foetus, family member, the general public. Risk communication is the open two-way exchange of information and opinion about risk, within a shared decision-making framework, which hopefully leads to better understanding by the patient and better decisions about clinical management by doctor and patient.[1] In the medical literature risk is generally defined in terms of numerical odds or probabilities, yet research has shown that patients find such terms difficult to understand. Moreover their understanding is likely to be affected by their age, educational level, health status and recent experience of illness.[2] The challenge, to be met by the learning sessions, is to enable health professionals to translate the language of risk into a format that a patient may understand.

Some definitions

It will probably be helpful to start the learning session with a discussion of how risk is conveyed. This will enable facilitators to pitch the subsequent activities at the right level. If the participants are fully conversant with the terms below, move onto the scenarios quite early in the session. It would be a good idea for there to be pre-session reading material to aid the opening discussion. The learners will not be able to communicate risk to patients if they do not understand it themselves.

When presenting figures relating to risk it is common to compare two groups of patients. The relationship between the two groups may be expressed in terms of absolute or relative risk. Often in the media, and indeed when sharing information with patients, it is not made clear whether absolute or relative risk is being expressed. An absolute difference is a subtraction; a relative difference is a ratio.[3] Because the choice of risk data may influence how big a difference seems, patients need to be aware of the distinction. Box 6.1 has a made up example to explain the terms, which could be adapted for use with patients.

Box 6.1   Absolute and relative risk

Consider the risk of going bald in a population of deep sea yodellers by the time they reach 60 years of age:

- with no treatment the absolute risk is 1 in 5 or 20%
- when using lotion X the absolute risk is 1 in 10 or 10%
- the *reduction in absolute risk* is 20 − 10 = 10% (0.1)
- lotion X reduces the absolute risk of baldness by 10%
- the *relative risk reduction* is the ratio of the two risks: 10%/20% = 50%
- lotion X reduces the relative risk of baldness by half (50%).

Without defining which risk is being used a doctor could tell a deep sea yodeller that lotion X reduces the risk of baldness by 10% or 50%. Obviously the second figure will sound a lot better and is likely to influence a patient's decision whether to use lotion X, especially if a possible side-effect of the lotion is loss of yodelling ability.

Absolute risk is expressed in terms such as 1 in 1000 or it may be given in percentage terms such as a patient has a 30% chance of having a stroke within the year if he does not reduce his blood pressure. The 30% may also be translated into: of ten people with the same risk factors as you, three will have a stroke within 1 year.

The *number needed to treat* (NNT) is a useful way of helping patients decide on whether to take medication by weighing up benefits compared to side-effects. The NNT is a figure showing how many patients must be treated before an adverse event such as stroke is prevented. NNT is calculated by the formula:

$$1 \div \text{absolute risk.}$$

So for our yodellers the NNT is $1 \div 0.1 = 10$. Ten yodellers must be treated with lotion X to prevent one case of baldness.

Scenarios for risk communication and informed consent

Communicating the risk of hormone replacement therapy (HRT)

Recent research findings concerning HRT have led to a change in the recommendations with respect to HRT prescribing. The data and information are changing all the time, but findings from the big studies provide a useful exercise for learners in communicating risk from research data. The learners should be given the data; it would not be realistic to expect them to remember it.

For:

Medical students, any doctor or nurse practitioner who has to communicate risk. It is also possible to use an adapted version for pharmacists.

Location

GP surgery or gynaecology outpatient clinic.

Patient

Monica Carter, a 51-year-old dressmaker.

Scenario for the SP

'I have been having hot flushes for the last 6 months. They are now interfering with my sleep and I am feeling tired a lot of the time. I am fairly sure that I am going through the change. My periods are becoming more infrequent, about every 6–10 weeks and are fairly light. I am otherwise in good health, happily married and enjoy my part-time job. I do not smoke. I take no medication and have no past medical history of note. My mother was diagnosed with breast cancer at the age of 64 and had a mastectomy. She died three years ago age 70 from the breast cancer. I have two brothers and no sisters.

I would like some treatment for the flushes and my best friend has recommended HRT. She thinks it is wonderful. However I have read that HRT can cause breast cancer and I would like more information. I also expect the doctor to discuss other risks of hormone treatment.'

Opening sentence
'I wonder if you can do anything about these hot flushes I'm getting. I think I am going through the change. A friend of mine recommended I ask about hormone treatment but I'm a bit worried about the risk of breast cancer.'

Information for the interviewer

You have not met Mrs Carter before. The medical records list two normal pregnancies and deliveries 25 and 22 years ago. Cervical smears are up to date, the last one was four years ago and normal. No other relevant notes.

Notes for the facilitator

This scenario can be run as a full consultation with information gathering about Mrs Carter's menstrual and sexual history, any risk factors for heart disease and family history, or the interviewer can be given all this information and asked to focus on giving the patient information about the risks of HRT. One learner could be given the relative risk data and one the absolute data. The group could then decide with the patient after the consultations, which are the easier figures to understand.

Risk data

The Million Women Study published in 2003 shows that in women taking combined HRT there is an increased risk in the following:[4]

* relative risk of breast cancer: 26%
* relative risk of ischaemic heart disease: 29%
* relative risk of stroke: 41%
* relative risk of pulmonary embolus: 213%

and the absolute risk for 10 000 women taking combined HRT each year, the number of extra cases of:

* breast cancer is 8
* heart attacks is 7
* strokes is 8
* pulmonary embolism is 8.

A patient requesting a PSA (prostate-specific antigen test)

This scenario is based on a challenging problem relating to screening and pre-test counselling. Learners will need to do some background reading on the subject. though risk data should be available on the day of the session so that they do not need to rely on memory.

For:

GP registrars, urology registrars, senior medical students.

Location

General practice or urology outpatient department.

Information for the interviewer

Your next patient is Derek Todd a 58-year-old garage owner.

Medical notes

Well man check three years ago. Non-smoker. Alcohol: 16 units (beer) per week. Vasectomy age 42. Parents both alive and well. Father has mild angina (age 82). Mother has arthritis (age 79). No relevant family history. BP 138/86 mmHg, BMI 26.

Scenario for the SP

'I am Derek Todd age 58, a physically fit garage owner.'

Opening statement
'I've been reading about the prostate test doctor and I was thinking I ought to have one.'

Continued

'I read about the test in the Sunday paper a few weeks ago and have been thinking about it. I know it is a blood test for prostate cancer. I also read that prostate cancer is quite common and that it is best picked up and treated early. I am not sure what my prostate is for but I think it has something to do with passing urine. I remember something about old men having to go to the toilet a lot and dribbling and that this can be cured by a prostate operation. I have no problems going to the toilet. I have a good stream, don't dribble and there is no pain. I occasionally get up at night to pass urine, usually when I have had a few beers. This is never more than once a night. As far as I know no-one in my family has had prostate cancer. My father is alive and fairly well at 82, though he takes some medication for angina. My mother has arthritis in her hips but is also doing well for 79. I have a younger brother age 55. I think I am fit for my age and when I had a check-up three years ago my BP was good. I could do with losing a few pounds but like my food. I have had no recent weight loss or gain.

I expect that the doctor will explain a bit about the test but I think it is a good idea to have it and expect that he/she will give me a form for the test. I would expect the result to be negative but you never know. My wife had a mammogram a few weeks ago and I think that this is a similar sort of thing for men, but a blood test rather than an X-ray. I expect information from the doctor and how this is discussed may affect my decision to have the test.

I will be surprised if the doctor tells me that I need a rectal examination: I would certainly want a good explanation for this.

I expect the doctor will:

- ask me why I want the test
- tell me a bit more about what the prostate does
- tell me more about the test
- give me some idea of my risk of prostate cancer
- tell me what might happen if the test is positive.'

Information to give the participants

Of 1000 men who are aged 50 years 136 will be diagnosed with prostate cancer before the age of 80 years, and 27 will die from the condition before the age of 80 years.[5]

The absolute risk of having prostate cancer is:

- 1 in 1000 at age 40–49 years
- 12 in 1000 at age 50–59 years
- 45 in 1000 at age 60–69 years
- 79 in 1000 at age 70–79 years.

Notes for facilitators

If the interviewer asks to do a rectal examination (DRE = digital rectal examination) tell him/her that this is normal, or give the SP a card with this information.

Box 6.2 lists the steps for informed decision making in relation to the PSA test and is a good framework for discussion after the consultation has been carried out.

> **Box 6.2   Informed decision making for PSA testing (adapted from Baade et al)[5]**
>
> ---
>
> - Explore the patient's concerns
> - Check understanding of what the prostate is, give further explanation as necessary
> - Explain the tests available
> - Explore the patient's risk of prostate cancer
> - Discuss the advantages and disadvantages of early detection
> - Identify the patient's preferences
> - Support the patient's choice

Ideas for development of this scenario

This scenario focuses on pre-test counselling in an asymptomatic patient. You may rerun the scenario with a patient in a different age group and/or change the medical history so that Derek's brother has recently been diagnosed with prostate cancer: this will double Derek's risk.[6]

If there is time run the follow-up consultation. Derek's result could be one of the following:

- 2.5 ng/ml (normal range cut-off)
- 4.5 ng/ml (just above the normal range)
- 15 ng/ml (above the normal range): this becomes a 'breaking bad news' scenario in that this is the result that Derek did not want to hear.

However a 2005 review of PSA testing in the USA has shown that there is no cut-off point of PSA with simultaneous high sensitivity and high specificity for monitoring healthy men for prostate cancer, but rather a continuum of prostate cancer risk at all values of PSA.[7] This may explain that while PSA testing has become common in the USA there has been no reduction in mortality from prostate cancer.

Discussing the risks of heart disease and stroke using risk calculators

Risk calculators are being increasingly used to help doctors and patients make decisions about when to treat high blood pressure and high cholesterol levels. But even before this point is reached patients are being offered 'well person checks' and these may involve discussion of whether to have a blood test to check the patient's cholesterol level.

There are therefore a sequence of scenarios that may be run at workshops on this topic (see Box 6.3) involving patients with different risk factors. As well person checks are often carried out by practice nurses, these scenarios are useful for running during primary care educational meetings to generate discussion about practice guidelines for screening and risk management. Participants may also wish to discuss how the sex of a patient affects management. How might the outcomes of the scenarios in Box 6.3 differ if the patient were male or female? Change the smoking status of the patients and discuss what happens. For the patients in Box 6.3 a risk calculator should be used as appropriate to assess the cardiovascular risk, and counselling then be given about management: whether an antihypertensive treatment should be started, whether a statin should be started.

Box 6.3   Patients attending for well person checks

- Age 40 years. No FH of heart disease. Non-smoker. BP 120/80 mmHg. Requests a cholesterol test.
- Age 55 years. Father died age 55 years of heart attack. Non-smoker. BP 140/90 mmHg. Requests a health check.
- Age 65 years. Father died age 75 years of stroke. Non-smoker. BP 150/90 mmHg. Requests a cholesterol test.
- Age 45 years. Smoker: 20–30 per day for 30 years. Father died in a road accident age 40 years. Mother is 80 years and has had a stroke. BP 164/96 mmHg. Requests a cholesterol test.
- Age 25 years. Father and uncle both had heart attacks in their mid-40s. Non-smoker. BP 120/80 mmHg.

Ideas for discussion

The New Zealand Cardiovascular Risk Calculator is a useful tool for assessing risk.[8] From the different patient details, blood pressure measurements and cholesterol levels, participants may calculate risk and discuss this with the appropriate patient. Absolute five-year cardiovascular risk and NNT data are available for the health professionals to convert into meaningful terms for patients.

Further information for discussion following scenarios

Patients are influenced by a number of factors when listening to information about risk (*see* Box 6.4).[9] The trust patients have in their doctors is thus of paramount importance in the process of risk communication.

Box 6.4   Influences on response to information about risk[9]

- The extent to which the source of information is trusted
- The relevance of the information for everyday life and decision making
- The relation to other perceived risks
- The fit with previous knowledge and experience
- The difficulty and importance of the choices and decisions

Patients understand different methods of presenting risk to varying extents.[10] Facilitators should pick up on ambiguous language used by learners as this is frequently misunderstood or misinterpreted. Words such as 'rarely', 'commonly', 'often', 'unlikely' and 'usually' mean different things to different people.

Framing is another way in which information is presented that has a bearing on patient choice. Positive framing involves describing outcomes in positive terms such as chance of survival, whereas negative framing concentrates on poor outcomes such as disability or dying.[11]

Informed and valid consent

The doctrine of informed consent is 'primarily American and relates to the amount of information that a patient should be given in addition to the broad nature requirement to avoid an action in negligence'.[12] When considering informed consent it is helpful for a doctor to consider the 'reasonable person standard' (also called the prudent patient test). This concept, established in the US in 1972, states that a doctor's decision about whether a patient should have been informed of a risk is based on whether a reasonable person in that patient's position would want to be informed.[13]

In England the courts apply the prudent doctor test that defines what a doctor should explain about an operation or other procedure as that information that would be disclosed by a responsible body of medical opinion; in other words what the medical profession agrees should be explained.[12] For consent for treatment to be valid, the conditions shown in Box 6.5 must be met. Discussion around the scenarios could focus on what happens if valid consent is not obtained; the doctor is at risk of being sued for negligence.

Box 6.5 Elements of valid consent

- The patient must have sufficient understanding to make the decision.
- The patient must consent to, or refuse, the treatment of his/her own free will with no duress or undue influence.
- The patient must have sufficient information about the proposed treatment.

Scenarios relating to valid consent should reflect the position and experience of the learners/participants. Possible simulations are shown in Box 6.6. When running a session around valid consent it is helpful to obtain copies of the local hospital's consent forms to use. A general practice may also have consent forms. If a practice does not have such forms, how does verbal consent differ from written consent, and what safeguards should be in place if only verbal consent is sought?

Box 6.6 Scenarios for informed consent

- Removal of benign skin lesion under local anaesthetic (LA)
- Biopsy or removal under LA of skin lesion that may be malignant
- First injection of Depo-provera
- Insertion of Mirena intra-uterine device
- Gastroscopy
- Female sterilisation
- Vasectomy
- HIV testing

Summary

Communication of risk is a relatively new development in consultations. It is one of the skills needed for shared decision making. Obtaining informed consent is an important process with many legal and ethical components.

References

1   Edwards AGK, Hood K, Matthews EJ et al. The effectiveness of one-to-one risk communication interventions in health care: a systematic review. *Med Decis Making*. 2000; **20**: 290–7.

2   Mazur DJ and Merz JF. Patients' interpretations of verbal expressions of probability – implications for securing informed consent to medical interventions. *Behav Sci Law*. 1994; **12**: 417–26.

3   American College of Physicians. www.acponline.org/journals/ecp/janfeb00/primer.htm

4   Million Women Study Collaborators. Breast cancer and hormone replacement therapy in the Million Women Study. *Lancet*. 2003; **362**: 419–27.

5   Baade PD, Steginga SK, Pinnock CB et al. Communicating prostate cancer risk: what should we be telling our patients? *Med J Aust*. 2005; **182**: 472–5.

6   Johns LE and Houlston RS. A systematic review and meta-analysis of familial prostate cancer risk. *Br J Urol Int*. 2003; **91**: 789–94.

7   Thompson IM, Ankerst DP, Chi C et al. Operating specific characteristics of prostate-specific antigen in men with an initial PSA level of 3ng/ml or lower. *JAMA*. 2005; **294**: 66–70.

8   www.nzgg.org.nz/guidelines/0035/CVD_Risk_Full.pdf (accessed 7 February 2006).

9   Alaszewski A and Horlick-Jones T. How can doctors communicate information about risk more effectively? *BMJ*. 2003; **327**: 728–31.

10   Say RE and Thomson R. The importance of patient preferences in treatment decisions – challenges for doctors. *BMJ*. 2003; **327**: 542–5.

11   Gigerenzer G and Edwards A. Simple tools for understanding risks: from innumeracy to insight. *BMJ*. 2003; **327**: 741–4.

12   Stauch M, Wheat K and Tingle J. *Sourcebook on Medical Law* (2e). London: Cavendish Publishing Limited, 2002.

13   Mazur DJ. Influence of the law on risk and informed consent. *BMJ*. 2003; **327**: 731–4.

Chapter 7

Breaking bad news

This chapter explores:

- different scenarios involving breaking bad news
- methods of communicating in emotional circumstances
- bad news relating to bereavement, test results and diagnosis of cancer
- dealing with relatives and confidentiality.

Bad or unfavourable news may be defined as 'any news that drastically and negatively alters the patient's view of her or his future'.[1] Medical students express concerns about 'breaking bad news' situations. They often want to learn how to do this before they have had practice of situations they are more likely to meet in their daily work on the wards and in the community. Students and junior doctors are rarely in a position, and really should not be expected, to break bad news. However they do need practice and experience in this area; working with SPs is one of the best ways to obtain a hands-on experience. More senior clinicians may also benefit from reviewing their communication and having an opportunity to express their feelings about these types of interactions.

Learning outcome for breaking bad news

- The ability to break bad news in a sensitive and empathic way

Scenarios for breaking bad news

Sudden infant death syndrome (SIDS)

This is an extremely distressing experience for all concerned. Unlike other examples of breaking bad news this death will not have been expected, therefore there is no way that a health professional can prepare a family to face what has happened. The bad news is usually given at the hospital where the baby has been taken and therefore a paediatrician is likely to be the doctor involved. But the family doctor is also an important figure in the aftermath of such a tragedy. The GP may have personal emotions or a sense of being unable to help that affects his/her role, and these can be explored during training sessions.

Additional learning outcomes

- Dealing with unexpected death
- Recognising one's own emotions
- Interacting with grieving family members
- Obtaining consent for a post-mortem

For:

Junior paediatric staff and other doctors who deal with breaking bad news.

Simulated mother and/or father

Mr and Mrs Johnson aged 28 and 26 years respectively. Their first and only child, Sam, aged 8 months has just died.

Location

Doctor's office in the local hospital.

Information for the parents

'We usually get up about 6.30 am. Sometimes Sam, who sleeps in a cot in our room, wakes us before this. This morning my husband Joe, Mr Johnson, woke first, got up, had a shower and made a cup of tea. He prepared Sam's bottle. As this was an at-home day for me, I enjoyed a few extra minutes lie in. Then I began to wonder why Sam wasn't making any noise. I got up and went over to the cot. Sam was on his back not moving, his lips looked blue. I was filled with a sense of dread. I picked him up and he was floppy and didn't make a sound. I remember screaming for Joe and shaking Sam a little bit. Then I put him on the bed and tried to give him mouth to mouth. Joe rushed in and immediately rang for an ambulance. The woman who answered gave us instructions about CPR (cardiopulmonary resuscitation)/heart massage over the phone. It seemed ages until the ambulance arrived. The paramedics took over and then took Sam to hospital. I went in the ambulance and Joe took his car and followed. At the emergency department they took Sam away and asked us to sit in this office. I was shaking and petrified. A doctor is coming to talk to us but I just want to see Sam. Where have they taken him?

Sam was born at 39 weeks' gestation and weighed 8 lb 7 oz. He has always been a healthy baby though he didn't sleep much in the first few months so Joe and I were often tired. However his sleep has been much better lately. He is growing well, smiling and sitting. He is up to date with his immunisations. I am a secretary at the local council and have been back working three days a week for the last month. Sam goes to a child minder on those days. He has had a snuffle the last few days but nothing to worry about. I took him to the GP three days ago and he was checked over: a mild cold the doctor said, and he certainly seemed better yesterday.'

Instructions for the doctor

You are about to see Mr and Mrs Johnson. Their son, Sam, was bought into A&E 30 minutes ago, but was dead on arrival. The paramedics had been working on him but he had not had a pulse for at least 15 minutes. He was pronounced dead 15 minutes ago. Mr and Mrs Johnson are in the office. You are fairly certain this is a case of SIDS but you need to ask them a few questions and inform them about the need for a post-mortem examination. You do not require their consent for this procedure, however you would like them to consent and be fully aware of the need for the examination.

Questions that the parents will ask

*   Can I see my baby now?
*   Why did my baby die?

- Was it my fault?
- I always put my baby to sleep on his back, so why did this happen?
- Would my baby have been in pain?
- Did my baby suffer?
- Was it something I did or didn't do?
- Was it because I didn't breast feed?
- What does SIDS mean? Is it the same as cot death? (if the doctor mentions this)
- What should I tell my friends?
- Does he have to have a post-mortem?

Notes for facilitators

This is a very emotional scenario and preparation of participants and debriefing is vital. While the Johnsons should give feedback in role, there may need to be a break of a few minutes or even more before feedback to allow the group to think about what they are feeling. If the 'doctor' is feeling upset, he or she will not be receptive to feedback. The facilitator needs to have a high awareness of the feelings in the room.

Pre- and post-test counselling for HIV (human immunodeficiency virus)

We do a lot of HIV testing and for most practitioners working with a low-risk population the majority of tests are normal. However pre-test counselling is important and mandatory in all situations, whether the patient has put him or herself at risk, or even if the test is required for a visa application.

Additional learning outcomes

- Pre-test counselling and preparation of patient for positive or negative result
- Eliciting a sexual history without being judgemental

Scenario 1: before the test

Opening line for the patient
'It's a bit embarrassing but I would like a check for sexual infections.'

Information for the patient
'I am Michael Stewart, a 35-year-old bookmaker. Two months ago I went to Thailand with my friend Ray for a wild bachelor holiday. I moved about the country and had sex with several girls I met in bars. I am not sure how many. I am not stupid and I used condoms on nearly every occasion but think I may have missed once or twice when I was very drunk. I have been back home for five weeks now. Yesterday Ray rang me in a panic. His girlfriend has just tested positive for Chlamydia and he thinks he must have given it to her following the Thai adventure. He has to see a doctor and thinks I should too. I have had no urinary symptoms at all: no frequency or burning. I am a fit man with no major illnesses or operations in the past. I have had no regular partner since splitting up with my last girlfriend six months ago. I have had sex on two occasions since returning home, both one-night-stands, but I wore a condom on each occasion. I don't know much about Chlamydia but I am also worried now about HIV and hope the doctor will suggest a test for that. I think the HIV test is a blood test, but I am not sure about other tests for sexual infections. I will freely admit to

Continued

what I have been up to, however I will be annoyed if the doctor asks me about sex with other men . . . I am definitely not gay.

   If the doctor asks me specifically what tests I want I will mention Chlamydia first. If the doctor doesn't suggest an HIV test I will have to ask for one myself.'

Information for the doctor/nurse

Your next patient is Michael Stewart age 35 years. He was last seen in the practice three months ago for a typhoid injection prior to travelling abroad. He was also given advice about malaria prophylaxis. His only other visit was for a shoulder injury five years ago.

Points for discussion

What should be covered before testing for any sexually transmitted infection and in particular before a test for HIV is requested? The group might brainstorm this question and should come up with a list similar to that shown in Box 7.1. The scenario could be run either in a GP setting or in a genitourinary medicine (GUM) clinic, and the possible differences in approach discussed.

Box 7.1   Pre-test counselling for HIV

- Elicit a sexual history and ask about any risk factors for STIs (sexually transmitted infections).
- Establish any past history of STIs and treatment.
- Are there any current symptoms of STI including rash, discharge, dysuria?
- Is there a specific risk for HIV?
- Give information about HIV infection and testing, including time taken for a test to become positive (window period of three months from the time of exposure until the test may become positive).
- Explain the meaning of a positive and negative test.
- Explore feelings relating to the possible test result.
- Explore what patient will do if the test is positive or negative.
- Discuss risk behaviour and how risk may be reduced.
- Give advice about local testing and when and where blood will be taken.
- Advise when the result will be back.
- Give advice about testing for other STIs and arrange testing.
- Discuss possible stress while waiting for results and how to manage this.
- Explore issues relating to confidentiality and contact tracing.
- Ensure that the patient's contact details are accurate.
- Arrange a follow-up appointment as appropriate.
- Check the patient's understanding of what has been discussed.
- Ask if there are any other questions or concerns.
- Write clear notes.

The group should also discuss what they feel about Michael's behaviour and how this might affect the way they interact with him. What would be the difference, if any, in their feelings if Michael was gay?

Scenario 2: after the test

Michael was tested for gonorrhoea, syphilis and Chlamydia. He tested positive for Chlamydia and has been treated. He had an HIV test immediately after his first consultation; this was negative. The HIV test was repeated three months after the unprotected sexual intercourse. This test is positive. He returns for the result.

Points for discussion

If Michael was prepared for a positive result by careful counselling during the first consultation, the doctor may build on this rapport and understanding. However Michael is going to be upset. The simulated patient will be able to discuss how it feels to be told he is HIV positive. There should be a discussion of what is to be covered in post-test counselling (*see* Box 7.2).

Box 7.2   Post-test counselling

- Ensure that the patient understands the significance of the test result.
- Encourage the patient to express his feelings by open questions and silences.
- Assess how the patient appears to have taken the positive result, e.g. grief, anger, denial.
- Explore what type of support the patient has in terms of family and friends.
- Discuss what type of support the patient would like from health professionals.
- Arrange appropriate follow-up with specialist HIV counsellors and support services.
- Go over the possible course of the condition.
- Discuss the need for safe sex practices.
- Explore again any possibility of transmission to sexual partners.
- Arrange medical referral.
- Discuss confidentiality of results and who the patient needs to tell.

Breaking bad news in relation to cancer

In the past, doctors tried to shield their patients from poor prognoses, even considering it inhumane or detrimental to patients to be honest about diagnoses.[2] The patient-centred approach and shared decision-making model encourage doctors to be more open when giving and sharing information. This openness and honesty is appropriate in most cases and follows the wishes of patients who have been shown to want to know if their diagnosis is cancer.[3]

While there are many occasions on which a doctor may need to break bad news, and many different types of bad news that this may be, the common scenario involves telling a patient that he or she has cancer. It is difficult to develop a true-to-life scenario as the bad news is rarely broken in isolation from the previous consultations, and depends very much on the existing relationship between the doctor and patient. When the doctor and patient know each other, the task, while daunting, should be less difficult. So the groundwork leading up to a possible poor prognosis begins at, or even before, a patient presents with symptoms that are potentially serious. The patient's anxiety regarding a possible diagnosis such as cancer may be elicited when he or she presents with sinister symptoms.

The doctor may thus be able to gauge how the patient will react to the possibility becoming reality, and have some idea of what and how the patient would like to be told. This doctor–patient relationship needs to be assumed in many of the scenarios as there is rarely time in the learning experience to build rapport; rapport that may take many interactions to develop fully.

Points for discussion

A breaking bad news scenario will lead to much discussion about the skills involved, the best way to tell patients, whether patients should always be told and how to deal with patients' emotions. However it is also important to explore the doctor's/learner's emotions. Like most work with simulated patients, the learner *becomes* the doctor and often feels sad and anxious following the scenario. Time is needed to de-role before feedback. But a skilful facilitated discussion of emotions will help learners to understand the pressures of their work and can lead to an exploration of self-care and how to deal with feelings once the patient has left.

Additional learning outcomes

* Ability to deal with one's own emotions: self-care
* Building rapport with a patient to ensure optimum care following diagnosis

Scenario for the SP

'I am David Fairfield, a 52-year-old musician. One week ago I came to see my GP because of a pain on the right side of my chest at the back. I had had this for about a week and it was steadily getting worse. I have not taken anything for it as I don't like to take painkillers; I prefer natural remedies. I thought it was probably muscular, but occasionally I had felt a bit short of breath. I have not had a cough. I have previously been fit and well. I get the occasional muscle aches and pains, and some joint twinges that I put down to age. I am fit and enjoy cycling. I have never smoked and enjoy a glass of wine about four times a week. My weight is steady. When I saw the doctor last week he/she examined my chest and said that there was possibly some fluid on my lungs. This surprised me, and I thought it might be some sort of infection, even though I don't smoke. However I didn't ask the doctor any more about this. The doctor sent me for a chest X-ray and I am coming back today for the results. I am a bit concerned but as I don't smoke I feel that there can be nothing seriously wrong. I have never married but I have been living with Sally an artist for the past three years. I have no children. My mother is still alive and well at 78, my father died of an accident when I was 20.

I want to know the X-ray results and expect to be told exactly what is wrong with me. I will push the doctor into giving a diagnosis if he/she is unclear. If the doctor says the word cancer I will be very upset and want to know where I got this from. If the doctor uses a word like malignancy, tumour, neoplasm, I will question this and what it means. I will stress I am a non-smoker and how could I have lung cancer?'

Notes for the doctor

David Fairfield age 52 years. Professional musician. Seen by yourself 1 week ago complaining of right-sided chest pain for 1 week. Non-pleuritic. The pain is becoming stronger and is now present all the time. No rash. Never had before. Slightly sob (shortness of breath). Non-smoker. No cough.

O/E pulse 80/min regular, BP 144/78 mmHg. Dull to percussion at right lung base extending up chest. Decreased breath sounds on right. No added sounds. Heart sounds normal. ?Pleural effusion ?Cause. For chest X-ray and review.

The chest X-ray report: there is a pleural effusion on the right side and shadows in both lungs suggestive of metastases. No evidence of primary lesion.

De-briefing

This is another difficult consultation. Feedback in role and the doctor being able to discuss his or her emotions in relation to breaking bad news are powerful tools for gaining the most from this learning experience. However before this may take place, the facilitator should check that the doctor and patient are able to carry on. There should be acknowledgement of the difficulty of the interaction. As well as direct discussion of the scenario, participants may be encouraged to discuss their own experiences of breaking bad news: what works well and what doesn't, how this is dependent on the existing doctor–patient relationship, how health professionals cope with such consultations and perhaps having to follow a 'breaking bad news' interaction with another emotionally charged consultation or one that is more mundane. Feedback from the patient may focus on how the patient feels in relation to the doctor's manner, the tone of voice, how the subject was broached, what may have made things better (or worse), and what the patient needs at the end of the consultation.

Skills for breaking bad news

There are several models for such interactions. Health professionals will find one that suits them, but this needs to be adapted for the individual patient and circumstance.

Baile and colleagues have developed a six-step protocol for breaking bad news, which they have called SPIKES (*see* Box 7.3).[4] Part 6 involves treatment decisions that may not be applicable in the GP setting, though there may need to be discussion of to whom and where to refer the patient.

Box 7.3   SPIKES protocol[4]

Step 1: SETTING up the interview
- Arrange privacy and make sure there will be no interruptions.
- Involve significant others as appropriate.
- Sit down.
- Connect with the patient: eye contact, touch.
- Advise the patient of the time you have available.

Step 2: Assessing the patient's PERCEPTION
- Use open-ended questions: 'What have you been told about your condition so far?'
- Gather information to explore the patient's perception of the situation.
- Explore ideas, concerns and expectations.
- Correct misinformation as necessary.
- This helps determine whether the patient is in denial.

Continued

Step 3: Obtaining the patient's INVITATION
- Find out how the patient would like to receive the information (this is a useful step at the time of ordering tests, so both doctor and patient are prepared for the way the results should be given).
- Gauge how much information the patient wants.

Step 4: Giving KNOWLEDGE and information to the patient
- Warn the patient that bad news is coming: 'Unfortunately I've got some bad news to tell you'.
- Break information into small chunks.
- Use appropriate language and check for understanding of each chunk of information.

Step 5: Addressing the patient's EMOTIONS with empathic responses
- Look out for the patient's emotional reaction.
- Identify the emotion e.g. anger, sadness.
- Identify the reason for the emotion, asking the patient if necessary.
- Make an empathic statement to acknowledge the emotion.

Step 6: STRATEGY and SUMMARY
- Present treatment options.
- Share decision making.
- Reach consensus.
- Plan follow-up.

Breaking bad news: dealing with concerned relatives

A common scenario is the well-meaning relative, often a daughter or son, who does not think the elderly parent will be able to cope with the diagnosis of cancer. Here there are issues relating to confidentiality, paternalism and bending the truth.

Additional learning outcomes
- Dealing with anxious relatives
- Maintaining confidentiality

Location

GP surgery.

Scenario for the SP

'I am Frances Parkinson, a 48-year-old teacher. My father Geoffrey age 82 has been undergoing some tests at his GP's for back pain and blood in his urine. He has just had an ultrasound scan of his bladder and kidneys and is due to return for the results tomorrow. I am staying with my father as it is the school holidays and I have made an appointment to see his GP today. I have not seen this doctor before but my father seems to like him/her. I have been reading up about the symptoms Dad has and I suspect that my father has bladder cancer, possibly with secondaries in his back (this seems to be a fairly common picture). I am going to ask the doctor not to tell my father he has

Continued

cancer, if indeed this is the case. I realise that the doctor will probably not be able to give me the test results but I do expect that he/she will be able to discuss matters in general terms. I also expect the doctor to be sympathetic to my viewpoint as I know my father better than anyone and can predict how he will react to bad news. My mother (his wife) died six months ago from breast cancer and she was in a lot of pain towards the end of her life. My father has not really recovered from his loss and I do not think he will cope with his own ill-health. He will probably give up altogether. I am also feeling rather low but won't show this to the doctor unless I am directly asked how I am feeling or how I am coping with all this upset.'

Information for the doctor

Your next appointment is Frances Parkinson, a 48-year-old lady, who is a temporary resident. You can tell from the computer screen that she is staying with Geoffrey Parkinson, an 82-year-old patient who presented a few weeks ago with painless haematuria and low back pain. His scan result shows a filling defect in the bladder and lumbar spine X-ray shows bony metastases. You know he is due to come in tomorrow for his results. You also remember that Geoffrey's wife died 6 months ago of metastatic breast cancer.

Points for discussion

* What can the doctor tell the daughter?
* How should the doctor react to being asked not to be completely open about the test results?
* Don't forget the daughter's needs: she is also receiving bad news in a roundabout way.
* Should the doctor suggest that the daughter accompanies her father for the consultation tomorrow?

A similar scenario may be used for hospital staff. In this case the patient will be an inpatient waiting for the results of tests and the daughter will ask to speak to one of the doctors or nurses looking after her father. How should the clinician respond to the opening gambit: 'Are my father's test results back yet?'?.

Summary

Breaking bad news is one of the most difficult tasks we face as health professionals. Practising the skills before having to perform such a task in 'real life' is a powerful tool to help professionals feel better prepared.

References

1 Buckman R. *How to Break Bad News: a guide for health professionals*. Baltimore: John Hopkins Press, 1992.
2 Oken D. What to tell cancer patients: a study of medical attitudes. *JAMA*. 1961; **175**: 1120–8.
3 Meredith C, Symonds P, Webster L *et al*. Information needs of cancer patients in West Scotland: cross sectional survey of patients' views. *BMJ*. 1996; **313**: 724–6.
4 Baile WF, Buckman R, Lenzi R *et al*. SPIKES – a six-step protocol for delivering bad news: application to the patient with cancer. *Oncologist*. 2000; **5**: 302–11.

Chapter 8

A selection of difficult interactions

This chapter explores a series of 'difficult' and intricate consultations for the more advanced clinician:

- request/demand for inappropriate medication
- working with patient's needs and wants
- communication through interpreters
- interaction with patients following a missed diagnosis
- dealing with a patient complaint
- the verbally aggressive patient
- complex medical problems.

Patients demanding inappropriate medication (benzodiazepines/methadone): a demanding and potentially aggressive patient

Learning objectives

- To experience an interaction with an aggressive patient
- To discuss strategies for dealing with aggressive patients
- To discuss strategies for dealing with patients demanding drugs
- To be able to apply communication techniques in a challenging situation
- To remember to explore each particular patient's story and not to judge on the basis of stereotyping
- To enable the discussion of similar real experiences and the emotions aroused

For:

General practice registrars because they are highly likely to be in this situation in practice, other junior doctors, doctors training to work within substance misuse clinics.

Patient

Andrew Brennan, age mid-30s. He is an alcoholic with a long history of substance abuse.

Location

General practice consultation (can be modified for emergency department). This patient has not been seen by this doctor before. He has been registered with the practice for 4 weeks but has not been seen by anyone yet. There are no records available.

This scenario is challenging as it is written. The patient may become aggressive depending on how the doctor interacts with the patient to address the patient's demands.

This scenario may be easily adapted for use with senior medical students, who may request such a scenario as a result of a consultation they have seen or a patient they have interacted with in the emergency department

Scenario for the SP

> 'I am Andrew Brennan. I am talking to this doctor in order to get as many benzodiazepines as possible (and any amount of methadone, as I know I can sell this on this street).'
>
> **Opening statement**
> 'I put out my hand to shake the doctor's hand [from the authors' experience no-one has declined to shake Andrew's hand]. Maintaining the doctor's handshake I will say: "I'm not here to take your time up doctor, I just want some of those benzos to tide me over".'

Andrew is under the influence of several substances (alcohol, tobacco, possibly cannabis). His speech is surprisingly quick and clearly demanding. He keeps eye contact. Andrew is wondering what effect he is having on this doctor: he is weighing him/her up.

What happens next depends on how the doctor responds and what he/she does.

Andrew Brennan's relevant history

Andrew is 32 years old and has a long history of alcohol and substance misuse. He is working class. His father was an alcoholic and was frequently violent at home. He has had no contact with his family since he left home as a teenager. Andrew has found employment mainly as a builder. He has moved frequently around the country as a result of having different jobs. He claims benefits as well as working. Andrew is currently living in rented accommodation with a woman who, he will claim, has drug-dependency problems and can't be trusted.

Andrew actually drinks three to four cans of Special Brew (8% alcohol) during the day, four to five pints in the pub. If he's with people who are smoking cannabis, he will. Usually later in the night he will search for heroin to smoke or methadone (he has never injected). He needs benzodiazepines 'to bring himself down'. He obtains his drugs on the street when he has cash; he also obtains temazepam and diazepam from GPs he sees around the country. He has been previously registered as a drug addict and has had methadone in the past from doctors. Andrew knows he can cheat on the 'swallow on site' rules (i.e. drugs are dispensed to the patient daily by a recognised pharmacist and the patient has to swallow them at the pharmacy and in front of the pharmacist; this is to try to prevent people taking away the drugs to sell).

How the scenario might unfold

- If the doctor is anxious and nervous Andrew will become more aggressive.
- If the doctor refuses to prescribe any treatment at all very quickly, he will shout and bang the desk or knock his chair over.
- If the doctor says he's calling the police, Andrew will threaten to burn the doctor's car.
- If the doctor is controlled and assertive, keeping possible worries internalised, and engages Andrew in the consultation by exploring what can be done for Andrew, Andrew will be more receptive.
- If the doctor relates to Andrew in a personal way in the early stages of the consultation, Andrew will accept this in order to get what he wants later.

Note

- As Andrew Brennan, the SP in role will use his intuition to gauge how the doctor is responding and will react accordingly to get what he wants.
- If the interviewing registrar/student is over-challenged in this scenario, the facilitator should ask Andrew Brennan to stop the consultation, but not come out of the role. This is often accompanied by a break in tension for the interviewer and the learning group, however the patient is not part of this break in tension and should just sit and stare at the floor, pull out a newspaper or fiddle with his fags or lighter etc *still in role*.

Notes for facilitators

- This is a difficult consultation and the 'doctor' may feel upset/angry/frustrated during and/or at the end. Debriefing is extremely important, as is stopping the consultation if you feel that the interaction is no longer educational.
- However, as this is a likely scenario in some format in real life general practice, it is a useful experience to act out in this less threatening situation than real life.
- During feedback, in role, Andrew may be asked to give his impression of the doctor's actions: what could the doctor have done to defuse any potential aggression? This is also something for the group to discuss, but Andrew's feedback is extremely important, and the validity of this depends very much on the experience of the SP taking the role.
- The scenario may also be used to look at the legal duty of doctors in prescribing in these instances, how they feel about 'drug seekers', safety within the surgery, whether it is possible to feel any empathy towards Andrew, and long-term strategies for managing drug seekers.

A variation for practice staff

Andrew presents at the practice reception demanding to see a doctor. There are no appointments apart from 'emergencies'. Andrew says it is an emergency. The receptionist role-plays his/her reaction and management of this situation. In this way receptionists are able to act out strategies for dealing with aggressive patients and feel more confident in their interactions with such situations.[1]

Patient with escalating and inappropriate (in doctor's view) need for strong analgesia

Learning objectives

- To discuss strategies for dealing with patients requesting certain types of drugs
- To be able to apply communication techniques in a challenging situation
- To remember to explore each particular patient's story and not to reveal judgemental behaviour due to stereotyping during the interview
- To enable the discussion of similar real experiences and the emotions aroused
- To explore the risk factors for patient behaviour and the role of the prescriber in addiction to analgesia

For:

GP registrars and senior medical students (possibly while on mental health attachments).

Patient

Sandra Patterson is a 44-year-old hairdresser.

Location

Patient presenting in general practice. Sandra has been registered with the practice for 4 years.

Medical records

With such a patient these would be quite extensive and the doctor may not have time to read them all before seeing Sandra, therefore just a summary is given:

History of back pain for 10 years. She has a repeat prescription for co-codamol (codeine 30 mg/paracetamol 8 mg) and receives 100 tablets every one month. She had her last prescription without being seen two weeks ago. She saw an orthopaedic surgeon three years ago: diagnosis mechanical lumbar back pain. Sandra also has difficulty sleeping and in the past has been given temazepam. Her last prescription for this was for 30 tablets × 10 mg three months ago. Two months ago she attended the local A&E department with 'renal colic' and was given an injection of pethidine. She was advised to see her GP for follow-up but this is the first time she has been back to the surgery since.

This is also a challenging consultation with a drug seeker, however Sandra becomes tearful rather than aggressive.

Scenario for the SP

'I am Sandra Patterson, a 44-year-old hairdresser. I have a lot of family problems at the moment and am hoping that the doctor will give me some tranquillisers to help the problem.'

Opening statement
'I look unhappy and avoid eye contact with the doctor at first. I say "I'm having real problems with my daughter and I don't think I can cope any longer".'

Relevant history
'I am married with two daughters aged 22 and 17. My older daughter is at university but still lives at home. She refuses to help in the house. She has a job as a waitress at the weekends and I think she spends all her wages on drugs; probably ecstasy and speed. I have noticed that she eats and sleeps erratically and her skin is often very spotty. She gets very aggressive and last night threatened me with a knife. The younger daughter has started to imitate her. She is still at school and is becoming very rude to me. My husband just wants a quiet life and won't interfere. He tells me to get on with it and sort it out. He goes out into the garden and reads in the shed. I can't sleep and can't concentrate on work. Two months ago my back pain got really bad and I went to Casualty at 3 am. They said I might have a kidney stone and gave me an injection which was wonderful. Maybe I will go back again to get another if I have a really bad night. The doctors at the hospital said I should see my doctor to arrange a kidney scan but I didn't as I reckon the pain was my back again. They gave me more of my painkillers, though I didn't say I was taking these regularly. I work three days a week in a salon but haven't felt able to go in this week. I usually work in spite of my back pain, so I reckon that I ought to get tablets otherwise I might not be able to work.

Continued

I need something for my nerves and hope the doctor will give me more temazepam, some diazepam and more painkillers. I have borrowed some diazepam from a friend a few times and I think it is really good: it helps me relax and stop worrying. I would like a stronger dose than 2 mg as I am sure that will be even better. I used to take diazepam for about five years when I started with back pain but the doctors at this surgery have never given me any.'

How the scenario might unfold:

- Sandra will tell the doctor about her family problems at great length if the doctor is receptive.
- She won't ask for a script at the start of the consultation but she will later on if the doctor does not suggest giving her one.
- She will ask for tablets, but will then ask for more to be put onto the prescription.
- She will become more emotional if the prescription is refused.
- She will deny seeking drugs from the hospital and will again become tearful so that her story of going to A & E does not make sense.
- If asked she will say she understands the risks of addiction with diazepam, but she was able to come off it before.
- She really needs something to help her: she will decline counselling or other forms of help.

Notes for facilitators

- Sandra's story about her family is real and the reactions of the 'doctor' and the group members may be explored to see how much they feel is true.
- This is a good case for exploring judgemental behaviour and stereotyping patients.
- It is useful to discuss how the group's feelings change from perhaps sympathy/ empathy/understanding at the beginning of the story, once Sandra begins asking for drugs.
- The scenario also may be used to discuss how patients are initially prescribed painkillers and tranquillisers, and how repeat prescriptions may be avoided.
- The group could discuss how they would feel if the patient's opening statement is: *'My back's bad again and I need some more painkillers'*.

Consultation with a non-English-speaking patient

We suggest this patient is a non-English speaking person but the main issue is that the health professional and the patient do not speak the same language.

Learning objectives

- To understand the communication barriers when interacting with non-English-speaking patients
- To explore ways of facilitating communication in such situations
- To experience working with interpreters
- To discuss who is appropriate to act as an interpreter
- To be culturally safe and aware

The patient is Arabic speaking, but this should be adapted according to whether there are SPs with other languages available. Recruiting SPs from a wide variety of ethnic and cultural backgrounds is helpful when working through these types of interactions.

For:

GP registrars, medical students and other health professionals who work with interpreters.

Patient

Shakira Akbar, a 33-year-old Sudanese refugee living in a local hostel with her husband Dappa and her 3-year-old daughter. She comes to the surgery with her husband. Shakira only has a few words of English. Her mother tongue is Arabic.

Location

General practice surgery.

Medical records

There are no medical records for this patient.

Scenario for the SP

'I am Shakira Akbar, a 33-year old Sudanese refugee living in a local hostel. I came to the UK six months ago as a political refugee with my husband Dappa, age 28, who was a business student in the Sudan. I have a 3-year-old daughter, Sameera. I speak very little English; Dappa's English is reasonable. I have been having heavy and painful periods for the last 9 months. The bleeding occurs every three weeks and lasts for up to 10 days. The pain is very bad and my husband has been buying me paracetamol. After the birth of my daughter I used the depot contraceptive injection but I last had this in the Sudan about one year ago (not sure of dates). I did not have much bleeding when using this. I have not been using contraception since. I feel very tired and I have lost some weight since the move. I want to sleep all the time but have to look after my daughter. My husband has been looking for a job and spends most of his time away from the hostel. I miss my sisters and mother who are still in the Sudan. I have not had any bleeding after sex.'

Information for Dappa (Shakira's husband)
'I have some understanding of English, enough for everyday conversation, however I feel uncomfortable talking about women's problems. I do not know what a cervical smear is. I am concerned about my wife. I would like more children in the future and wonder why she hasn't become pregnant in the last few months, as we have been using no contraception.'

Opening statement (by the husband)
'My wife is very tired and is always bleeding.'

Points for discussion

The discussion relating to this scenario can take many directions and involves several tasks (*see* Box 8.1). Overall the facilitator should encourage the group to think about the needs of the patient and the importance of involving a trained interpreter in future consultations with Shakira.

Box 8.1 The case of Shakira

- Establish how much English the patient both speaks and understands.
- Establish how much the 'interpreter' speaks and understands.
- Is the patient comfortable with her husband (or other relative) acting as interpreter?
- Is the doctor comfortable with the husband (or other relative) acting as interpreter?
- Elicit a medical history.
- How much is the social history important? How much of the personal circumstances of the patient should be explored, including the reason for leaving her own country?
- What cultural aspects of the patient's life and beliefs impact on the medical problem and its likely management?
- Does Shakira wish to become pregnant?
- Is contraception required?
- What are the barriers to performing an intimate physical examination?
- Screening: discuss cervical smears and if and when the patient last had one.
- How may the doctor involve an Arabic-speaking interpreter?
- How does the doctor feel about the lack of communication?
- How does the doctor know if his/her words and the patient's words are being conveyed accurately?
- Ensure that all parties concerned understand the confidential nature of the consultation.

If it is possible the consultation should be re-run with an Arabic interpreter present. (The scenario could be rewritten to reflect the availability of an interpreter.) Interpreters should work in such a way that both the effect and meaning of words and phrases are conveyed, and ideally should have relevant cultural knowledge and an appropriate professional background.[2]

This scenario is based on a real case. However the patient's voice can only be conjectured unless the communication skills team are able to talk to refugee patients to hear their own voices and stories. Stories of refugees told in the first person are often published in books and magazines and these may be adapted for communication skills work. Scenarios may be written which have a focus on patients who have been tortured or abused in their home countries. Such consultations are extremely distressing, but hopefully helpful in the long term for both future patients and health professionals.

Consultation following a mistake on the part of a doctor or health professional

Everyone makes mistakes. Many of these are trivial: calling a patient by the wrong name and having the wrong set of notes; forgetting to call a patient as promised with normal test results. Some are more serious and a few may have life-threatening consequences. In the past, doctors were advised never to admit that they had made a mistake and, if patients complained, not to answer them until legal advice had been sought. The rising interest in patient safety issues and public awareness of how many adverse events and critical incidents occur in hospitals and primary care has led to a more transparent system, in which mistakes and near misses are discussed, often with patients being involved. Patients often complain about their care in order to find out what exactly went wrong. When health professionals are honest and frank, there is less likely to be a formal procedure. However how often do we practise apologising to patients?

Learning objectives

* To acknowledge that mistakes occur
* To have strategies for dealing with patients following mistakes
* To be able to apologise to patients
* To discuss feelings relating to such interactions and how these may be dealt with
* To explore patients' wants and needs with regards to apologies and knowing what went wrong

For:

GP registrars and GPs. May be adapted for hospital doctors.

Patient

Moira Beeston is a 68-year-old retired clerk. She has been a widow for five years.

Location

General practice.

Scenario for the SP

'My name is Moira. I live by myself in a retirement flat. My husband died five years ago of a heart attack. A few months ago I noticed a lump near the middle of my chest just to the side of my breast bone. I didn't think it was in my breast but it worried me. I had also noticed that my voice had been going a bit hoarse for a few weeks as well. I went to see my GP but she was away on holiday for a few weeks so I saw a new doctor who I thought was quite young. However she was very attentive. I asked her to look at the lump. She seemed more concerned with my voice and the fact that I smoked. She examined my throat, chest and breasts. She said that she thought the lump was on one of my ribs and that I ought to see a throat specialist about my voice. She also arranged for me to have a chest X-ray. A week later she called me up and said the X-ray was OK and that I had an appointment at the hospital in a week's time. I saw the doctor at the hospital who told me I had chronic laryngitis and a small nodule on my vocal cord. This was removed and luckily it was benign. However I was still worried about the lump in my chest. I went back to see my own GP who referred me to a breast surgeon and a few weeks later I had a mastectomy for breast cancer. I have been feeling fairly angry with the first doctor, and my son thinks I should make a complaint. I am not sure whether to do this. This morning the doctor rang me and asked if he/she could come and talk to me at home.'

Information for the doctor

A few months ago you saw Moira, whom you had not met before. She was worried about a lump in her chest but you noticed that she had a hoarse voice and asked her about this. You also noted that she was a 20-a-day smoker. You examined her chest and breasts and felt that the lump was on one of her ribs. You arranged a chest X-ray and referral to an ENT surgeon. The X-ray was normal. Last week your partner said that Moira has just had a mastectomy for breast cancer. You decided to go to see Moira at home once she was discharged from hospital.

Medical records

Age 68. c/o small lump just on right side just lateral to sternum, noticed a few days ago. Also has hoarse voice for a few weeks. No URTI (upper respiratory tract infection), smokes 20/day since age 20. No sore throat. No weight loss. No FH of cancer. No cough. O/E: throat looks NAD, breasts no masses, no lymph nodes, 2 cm lump, fixed, appears to be on rib. For chest X-ray and referral to ENT specialist. CXR (chest X-ray) normal. Patient rung with result and date of urgent ENT appointment.

Notes for facilitators

Before interacting with the patient, the group should discuss their feelings and suggest ways in which to consult with Moira. Some of the participants may have been in similar situations in respect to less than perfect management of patients in the past, and this scenario is very difficult and challenging. I would not suggest starting the consultation without a briefing unless the participants are experienced practitioners. With this scenario it will probably be the doctor who starts the interaction by expressing his or her own reason for the home visit, an interesting development in itself compared to the majority of consultations.

   After the consultation the doctor may need to come out of role for a while before feedback. It is important to evaluate fully how the participants are feeling and ensure that the group is still able to learn. The SP also needs adequate support and training before and after the scenario.

Points for discussion

*   What do the group feel that doctors should do in cases where mistakes have been made?
*   If the group is working well together, participants may share mistakes they have made in the past and how they dealt with these.
*   The group may also wish to discuss how mistakes have been dealt with by their seniors and the administration.
*   The patient's input is important for this discussion: how does she feel, how would she have felt if the doctor hadn't come to see her?
*   Should one always admit one's mistakes?
*   What if there is no adverse outcome or the mistake is rectified before any harm comes to the patient (a near miss)?

Variations on the scenario

*   Run the consultation between Moira and her usual doctor after the diagnosis of breast cancer is made.
*   Run the consultation between the two doctors. How should Moira's usual doctor tackle her colleague's mistake?

- Replay the home visit with Moira's son also present.
- Run a consultation between the doctor and Moira's son.

Other possible scenarios relating to mistakes

- Doctor or nurse gives patient a wrong injection (e.g. Depo-medrone instead of Depo-provera)
- Doctor gives patient a wrong prescription as he/she had the wrong set of computer notes on screen for another patient with same name
- Pharmacist rings doctor because too high a dose of a drug has been written on a prescription

Dealing with a formal complaint from a patient

Learning objectives

- Communication skills for dealing with distressed patients and relatives
- Ability to deal with complaints in an empathic and professional manner

For:

This scenario is for people who deal with patient complaints and who interview the patients or their relatives in respect of these. These may be senior doctors, hospital managers or practice managers.

Scenario for the SP (a relative)

'I am Jodie Simpson a 33-year-old female who works as a student feedback co-ordinator at the local university. I am happy and respected in my workplace. I carry out voluntary extra duties such as organising staff coffee mornings and small parties to celebrate their birthdays. I help improve staff morale in difficult times by asking staff to buy small gifts which they exchange with each other. I understand the importance of feedback in staff development and ensuring that students have the best learning experiences.

I report to senior management about issues arising from student feedback. In the work environment I will openly criticise and question staff and their actions or apparent lack of work ethic. I have made several complaints against poorly functioning staff. One complaint was a formal one.

My partner is Gordon, age 40. We have been living together for eight years. Gordon has four children from a previous relationship. While there are tensions at home on the whole we are a happy family.

Gordon has a history of bowel problems, ulcerative colitis and rectal bleeding and was referred to the university hospital for a colonoscopy by his GP. I went to the surgical clinic with Gordon to support him and also for this reason: patients are asked to bring somebody with them since a sedative painkiller is given to the patient in order for the procedure to be undertaken, and this might render 'the patient unable to recall discussions with the doctor', as the information booklet reads.

We had been downplaying our anxiety about the operation by joking about Gordon having an aerial stuck up his bottom and needing surgery to get better reception on the car radio. We had to wait a while after the colonoscopy for the doctor to come to talk to us. The doctor's facial expression was stern and we thought him a bit standoffish.

Continued

These are the concerns that I have about our treatment and which I have made a complaint about:

1 After surgery while waiting for the discussion Gordon told me that a nurse or anaesthetist (not sure which) explained that he would be given a general anaesthetic as his procedure involved pumping gas into his intestines which is uncomfortable for the patient. This advice was unexpected because the patient information form (obtained from the surgeon's office the week before) said a sedative painkiller would be given.

2 Before the colonoscopy the 'surgeon' introduced himself to Gordon only. Neither Gordon nor I had met him before. This lack of courtesy upset me as I thought myself part of the team.

3 Gordon tried to downplay the significance of the procedure saying that it was only precautionary as his father had had bowel cancer. The doctor dismissed this comment and walked off without closing the interview. I was a little disturbed at this.

4 Gordon remembers that he saw the doctor looking at a monitor, and feeling the doctor remove the colonoscope at the end of the procedure.

5 Gordon was wheeled to the recovery area and opened his eyes when a nurse put an oxygen mask on him. The nurse said 'Oh you're awake' as though she thought Gordon was still under anaesthetic.

6 In the recovery area a man in a surgical gown walked towards Gordon and me, and called for Gordon Bailey. Gordon waved the doctor over. He asked if I was Gordon's wife and I told him I was his fiancée. The doctor then ignored me and did not address me again.

7 The doctor handed Gordon an envelope for his GP and a list of what patients can and cannot do after an operation. He told Gordon that the operation had been successful as he had removed a couple of polyps. The doctor said he "would see him in another 5 years for another colonoscopy" and then turned around and walked off. He did not explain about the polyps.

8 Gordon told me that the doctor was abrupt in his speech. I thought he was arrogant and felt this was reinforced by the doctor's attitude. His tone of voice was stern and abrupt.

9 The staff of the hospital kept calling me Mrs Bailey even though Gordon's patient information sheet listed me as Jodie Simpson.'

Note for facilitators

This is a complicated scenario. The interviewer should be given the numbered points above as the letter of complaint.

Points for discussion

- Why do patients make complaints?
- How should they be dealt with?
- What further action should be taken with regard to the above scenario?

A verbally aggressive relative with unreasonable demands

Learning objectives

- Ability to manage unreasonable demands from a patient with tact and empathy, and without becoming too emotional
- Strategies for dealing with patients who threaten to make unjustified complaints

For:

GP registrars and newly qualified GPs, practice nurses.

Location

General practice.

Information for participants

It is the fortnightly well baby clinic at your surgery. This clinic is for developmental checks and childhood immunisations. It is practice policy for the attending doctor not to see ill mothers or babies: these will be seen at the afternoon surgery after the clinic as there is no time set aside for this. The next baby to be seen is Joshua Smith, age 3 months, for his second injections. His mother is Kylie Johnson, a 16-year-old single parent. She comes with her mother 40-year-old Annette Johnson. Annette is well known in the practice for frequently demanding appointments and often not turning up. The receptionists say she often shouts at them if they can't give her what she wants. She is always asking for painkillers for various aches and pains. In contrast, Kylie is a quiet girl and seems to be coping fairly well under the circumstances.

Joshua was born by vaginal delivery at 39 weeks' gestation and weighed 3.2 kg. Kylie's postnatal examination at 8 weeks revealed no abnormalities. She is on no contraception.

Scenario for the SP: Annette

'I am 40 and divorced. I am here at the well baby clinic with my daughter Kylie and the baby. Joshua is a lovely boy but I am worried about Kylie. She has been bleeding almost constantly since the delivery, not a lot but enough to wear towels. I am going to ask the doctor/nurse about this. I intend him/her to examine Kylie and sort out the problem. If the doctor/nurse won't look into this problem I will be very angry and threaten to make a complaint.'

Opening statement
'While we're here with the baby I want you to do something about Kylie's bleeding.'

Note

If an SP as Kylie is available, the doctor/nurse may begin to elicit a history, but this is not the aim of the scenario. The scenario should be introduced with a clear statement of the practice policy regarding the conduct of the well baby clinic. Once the doctor or nurse reminds Annette of this policy Annette will become more assertive and then more verbally aggressive: I demand that you sort this out, if you don't I will take her to casualty, I will make a complaint, who do you think you are etc.

Notes for facilitators

Only Annette needs to be present for this consultation. The group may discuss at the end what practices may do about such verbally aggressive patients, particularly in view of the receptionists' reports about Annette's behaviour.

* What justifies removing a patient from a practice list?
* What is the mechanism for this?
* What about the rest of the family?

- What might be the underlying cause of Annette's behaviour?
- How should this be explored?

A patient with multiple problems and a mistrust of doctors

Learning objectives

- Strategies for building rapport with patients who do not trust doctors
- Dealing with a patient with multiple and complex health problems

For:

GP registrars and GPs.

Location

General practice.

Information for the doctor

The next patient is Steve Morgan, a 65-year-old retired farm worker. He has seen all three of the other doctors in your practice over the last three years, as well as two gastroenterologists. He has been complaining of abdominal pain, mainly in the right side, sometimes under his ribs, sometimes in his iliac fossa. He has had the following investigations in this time:

- gastroscopy: normal
- sigmoidoscopy: normal
- ultrasound of the liver, gallbladder, kidneys, bladder: normal
- computed tomography (CT) of the abdomen: normal
- porphyria screen: normal.

He has been tried on various medications with no success. During this time he was diagnosed with type 2 diabetes and started on glipizide. Six months ago he saw the diabetes educator, who advised him about diet and checking his own blood sugar.

Recent results:

- BP: 150/90 mmHg
- BMI: 31
- haemoglobin A1c (HbA1c): 10 mmol/l.

Scenario for the SP

'I am Steve Morgan. I have never been married. I used to work on a farm but have now retired and I am renting a flat near the surgery. Three years ago I was fit and healthy. Then I felt something burst under my ribs on the right side. It felt like fluid running down inside me. There was nothing to see on the outside. I am sure something burst. Since then I have had this almost constant stomach pain on the right side. Sometimes it goes away for an hour or so. I have seen loads of quacks about this and had lots of tests but they say they can't find anything. I have been put on all sorts of tablets, but I don't think the doctors know what they are doing. My bowels tend to be a bit constipated but that has always been the case. I have put on weight since I stopped working. I enjoy a few beers, but this pain has made me reluctant to go out. Two years ago I got put on some new pills and have been taking them on and off. I had to see a

Continued

woman about my diet. She told me to lose weight. But nothing has helped the pain. I am seeing this new doctor today. Perhaps this one will be able to do something.'

Opening statement
'I hope you are better than the other quacks I have been seeing. What can you do about my stomach pain?'

Notes for facilitators and the SP

Steve has been diagnosed with diabetes but he will say he didn't know this . . . no-one told him. They told him the pills were for the pain. He hasn't changed his diet and he certainly hasn't bought a machine to check his blood sugar.

This is a complex interaction. See how far the doctor gets in a standard 10-minute consultation.

Points for discussion

- How should the doctor handle criticism of his/her colleagues?
- How should Steve's problems be prioritised? What are his priorities? What are the doctor's?
- How may the doctor build up rapport with Steve?
- What explanation should be given in regards to his abdominal pain and his diabetes?
- What emotions does the doctor feel during the consultation?

Summary

This chapter has presented a whole bunch of difficult cases, but the type of interactions that we meet every day. They should generate a lot of discussion. Don't forget the patient's voice in such discussions. Don't let the health professionals do all the analysis.

References

1 Thistlethwaite JE, Pierce B and Martin A. Handling aggression: report of a multidisciplinary workshop. *Education for General Practice*. 1998; **9**: 452–5.
2 Robinson L. Intercultural communication in a therapeutic setting. In: Coker N (ed). *Racism in Medicine*. London: King's Fund, 2001, pp 191–210.

Chapter 9

Communication between health professionals

This chapter explores:

- telephone interactions
- interactions between junior staff and senior staff
- doctors as patients
- tackling poor performance
- whistleblowing
- interprofessional interactions.

Communication skills training has typically concentred on the interaction between health professional and patient. However in the course of a day a health professional will interact with many people other than patients. Senior clinicians may not only be in charge of a clinical team but may also be responsible for teaching junior staff both within and without their own disciplines. Chapter 10 will look at the more formal interactions between professionals and teaching, while this chapter looks at day-to-day communication issues.

In these scenarios we do not have 'simulated patients' as such but rather 'simulated doctors' or 'simulated health professionals'. The principles of working are the same.

Box 9.1 lists possible interactions that may be simulated (thus written communication is omitted). The scenarios may require the group participant acting as interviewer or subject to role-play.

Box 9.1   Interactions between health professionals

HP–HP (same profession) e.g. doctor–doctor
- Case discussion
- Handover
- Seeking or giving advice
- Telephone referral
- Appraisal and mentoring (*see* Chapter 10)
- Treating a doctor as a patient
- Informal positive feedback
- Informal 'negative' feedback to a junior

HP–HP (different profession) e.g. doctor–physiotherapist
- Telephone referral
- Seeking or giving advice

Continued

- Handover
- Case discussion

Running/chairing meetings
- Facilitating a small group educational meeting
- Practice meetings
- Committees
- Whistleblowing

Telephone referrals

Doctors seem to spend a long time on the phone arranging referrals, in particular on those occasions when a GP wants to admit a patient to hospital. Yet such communication, in our experience, is rarely taught. Hospitals have different systems of accepting patients: some have an admitting ward and the doctor speaks to a senior nurse, others admit only through the emergency department, while in yet others the GP speaks to the doctor-on-call for the relevant specialty. The skill in these situations is to be succinct and concise. Experienced GPs may get exasperated having to deal with junior doctors who question their decision to admit a patient.

Learning objectives

- Ability to present a case requiring admission in a concise and succinct manner
- Telephone etiquette

For:

Senior medical students and junior GP registrars.

Location

Patient's home or after-hours centre.

Notes for the facilitator

This scenario would work best if one of the participants were able to describe an occasion when he/she wanted to admit a patient and there was a problem with the admission process. The person responsible for admissions could be played by the simulator or one of the other participants. The latter would be particularly interesting if the group comprised a mix of registrars from both the community and hospital. In the case of medical students, they may be able to recall an occasion from their general practice attachments when the GP wanted to admit a patient and what transpired. Otherwise the following scenario could be used.

Scenario

For the participant
You have just seen a 26-year-old woman with right iliac fossa pain, fever and nausea. You have made a diagnosis of pelvic inflammatory disease (PID), and in view of the severity of

her symptoms you think she needs admission for a gynaecological assessment. You speak to the on-call gynaecology senior house officer.

Simulated doctor or group participant

A GP wishes to admit a patient with right iliac fossa pain. You need to be convinced that this is not a surgical case. If any pertinent details are missing you will decline to accept the patient. You may become quite abrupt if you feel the doctor is trying to 'hoodwink' you without a full history and examination.

Note for facilitators

Give the participant the patient's name and age. But he/she has to be able to convey the symptoms and signs of PID in order to 'convince' the admitting doctor that this is a gynaecology case. This means that the participant needs some knowledge in this area, as would be the case for a GP registrar. The group may also assist in discussing the likely presentation.

Points for discussion

The doctor/student must elicit a careful history and perform a relevant examination, as well as be able to convey a summary of these to the admitting doctor. Telephone etiquette and the professional way to talk to a colleague on the phone should be explored. If there is a mixture of participants in the group, both hospital and community, the difficulties facing both sets of doctors can be discussed, e.g. why it is difficult to perform a full examination in a patient's home, living with uncertainty, tiredness, what precipitates rudeness in some professionals etc.

Doctors as patients

Learning outcome

* Protocol for dealing with doctors as patients

For:

Junior doctors, ideally a mixed group of hospital and GP registrars. The scenario may be run as a role-play with two participants acting as the GP and the hospital doctor respectively. Or a simulated doctor may take the role of the second doctor. The scenario may be changed to reflect the specialty of the participant playing the patient.

Location

GP surgery.

Scenario

Doctor 1
'I am a newly qualified GP working in a small town. I recognise the name of my next patient as the same as one of the local cardiology specialists.'

Doctor 2
'I have been a cardiology specialist for 2 years. I have previously been in good health and am on no medication. I am a non-smoker but drink about half a bottle of wine five evenings a week. I used to exercise regularly, working out and jogging three times

---

Continued

a week, but in the last six months the rising workload (due to holidays and being the only cardiologist in town) and getting late home most nights means that I rarely do any exercise during the week. I try to walk five miles at the weekend but don't always manage it. In the last two months I have been getting intermittent chest pain that I have self-diagnosed as indigestion and I admit I have written myself a prescription for omeprazole. However the pain is now more frequent and seems to occur more when I am stressed. I am concerned that it is cardiac. I did ask one of my hospital colleagues for advice at the end of a meeting but he said it sounded like reflux to him. I can't really do an ECG for myself but I did get my cholesterol checked and it is 6.6 mmol/l. My father had an MI aged 62 but is still alive, and my mother is fit and well. I am embarrassed seeing this doctor. I didn't register with a doctor when I moved here two years ago so this is my first visit. I wanted to see one of the older doctors but they were booked up so I am seeing the most junior partner. I expect an examination and reassurance, but depending on what the doctor says I might want to be referred to a cardiologist in the city.'

Opening statement
'I just want some advice about my indigestion and a bit of a check-up.'

Points for discussion

- Protocol for dealing with a colleague
- Corridor consultations (e.g. the cardiologist asked a colleague for advice at the end of a meeting)
- How does each doctor feel about the consultation?
- Should the way the GP consults change because this is another doctor?
- What different outcomes are there for this consultation?
- Doctors having a GP

Resources

Refer to the British Medical Association (BMA) guidelines for sick doctors.[1] The guidelines are also the policy of the General Medical Council (GMC). The clear message is that doctors should not treat themselves or their families, and that all doctors should be registered with a GP. As with all other patients, the responsibility for overall care and continuity of treatment for doctors and their families should rest with their GP. Referral for consultant advice or care should be made through the GP. Furthermore, doctors should not prescribe for themselves anything other than over-the-counter medication.

Speaking to a colleague about perceived poor performance

Often in daily practice health professionals come across examples of what they perceive as poor performance or 'bad medicine' from a colleague. This might be a one-off incident involving a usually well-respected clinician. However the health professional who comes across the behaviour feels that he/she should bring it to the attention of the colleague, in order to ensure that it does not happen again, or to clarify what has in fact gone on.

Learning outcomes

- Ability to discuss perceived poor performance with a colleague
- Giving feedback to a colleague

This scenario is built upon the case of Sandra Patterson, the hairdresser from Chapter 8. Sandra has been seeing Dr M on a regular fortnightly basis to receive her prescriptions for analgesia and benzodiazepines. Her records are flagged that she should only see Dr M for these drugs. Dr M goes away on holiday for three weeks. Dr M has only given Sandra a two-week supply of medication. Sandra therefore has been to see Dr N. Dr N is angry that he/she has been put in the position of prescribing for Sandra without knowing anything about her case. Moreover there does not seem to be a management plan in Sandra's notes dealing with how her obvious addiction to these drugs is being managed. Dr N feels at the least that Dr M should have discussed Sandra's case at a practice meeting to ensure the doctors and nurses know about her. Dr M is normally an excellent GP. Dr N feels that he/she should discuss Sandra with Dr M and say that the incident was unsatisfactory.

Both Drs M and N can be played by GP registrars or GPs. Or Dr M can be played by a briefed simulated doctor. If there is a simulated doctor, the interaction could be run through twice. On the first occasion Dr M is open to Dr N's suggestions that the case was not handled well; on the second Dr M responds as if he/she feels that Dr N should mind his/her own business. The discussion should focus on the feelings of both doctors. How do participants feel about approaching a colleague in this way? What strategies may be used? What should happen if Dr M will not listen to the colleague's feedback?

The doctor with problems

A common examination or interview question is what to do about a colleague who is suspected of having a mental health problem including alcohol or drug abuse. Speaking of this in the abstract is difficult as one has to think of the legal and ethical issues arriving from such a case as well as the personal ones. Communication with the affected health professional is something that should be discussed, and working through a scenario with a simulated professional is a good way of rehearsing strategies. To start with we will consider the case of two doctors.

Learning outcomes

- Ability to broach a difficult topic with a colleague
- How to handle a colleague's perceived medical problem

Scenario

Doctor W (group participant)

'I have been working as a GP principal in this practice for 3 years. I am the junior of three doctors. Six months ago one doctor left to go overseas and we haven't been able to replace her yet. The senior doctor (X) has been working in this small town for over 30 years and is full of experience and knows most of the practice patients very well. He is looking forward to retirement though says he may stay on in a part-time capacity. None of us can really see him leaving. The middle doctor (Y) is in his 40s. He has been here for 15 years. While I get on really well with Dr X, I find him somewhat old-fashioned in his approach to patients. I have never warmed to Dr Y, who can be abrupt to the staff. However the patients seem to like him. In the last few months Dr Y has been even more brusque than usual and seems to find fault with everything. Recently he has started coming in a few minutes late for surgery and has been really unpleasant

---

Continued

to the receptionists when they ask him to see extra patients. He isn't as tidily presented either, and I'm sure he wears the same shirt for several days at a time. One of the nurses reckons he is having marital problems. She also told me that one morning in the treatment room he seemed to smell of alcohol, though I haven't noticed that myself. However a few of his patients have started coming to see me and Dr Y does seem to be making some odd clinical decisions. I would say he seems depressed. Perhaps it is the extra work we all have to do. I mentioned my concerns to Dr X but he said he hadn't noticed anything odd and that I should speak to Dr Y about my concerns myself.'

Doctor Y (simulated doctor or group participant)
'I am really fed up at the moment. The petty concerns of the patients are irritating me. The worried well and the moaning women: I really need a break. I have been seeing twice as many patients a week since that doctor left earlier this year, and the other two don't seem to be doing as much. On top of that my wife is always complaining about things, she thinks we should move to the city and get out more. She seems to be spending a lot of time with her friends and is often away at weekends. Often I can't find an ironed shirt in the house. My kids are always wanting stuff and I never seem to have any spare cash. I hate getting up in the mornings and can't get to sleep at night. Sometimes I have a few glasses of whisky before I go to bed and I have also taken some sleeping tablets so I can get a few hours' sleep. I'm sure things will settle down soon. I don't need any help. I'll sort this out myself. I am registered with a GP on the other side of town but haven't seen him for several years.'

Notes for facilitators

This is a familiar story: the burnt out doctor working in a practice during a crisis due to being one doctor down. The task of the junior partner is to help Dr Y see he has a problem and then discuss together ways in which he could be helped; in particular Dr Y should be advised to see his GP. Discussion after the scenario could explore several issues:

* Dr W may be torn between being Dr Y's partner and acting as a proxy GP.
* If Dr W suggests that Dr Y takes time off, the practice workload will go up yet again.
* How to broach the issue with Dr Y, avoiding a corridor consultation-type scenario.
* Who else is available to help?
* How is Dr Y getting hold of sleeping tablets?
* Are patients at risk?
* What is Dr X's role in all this? Should he be allowed to shrug off any responsibility?

Variations

This scenario has been written with a fairly low-key story. It could be replayed with variations still concerning Dr Y. For example he may start drinking more heavily and being verbally aggressive to staff. A patient may make a complaint about his behaviour. His drug use may escalate. Note that Dr Y may be male or female. The location could also be a hospital.

Another angle is to have Dr Y's behaviour occurring in a staff member, for example a practice nurse. Here issues relating to employment law and when to issue informal and formal warnings are important.

Whistleblowing

Whistleblowing is defined as 'to bring an illicit activity to an end by informing on [the person responsible]'.[2] While within the NHS most whistleblowing involves raising concerns about a process or system rather than an individual, the process of whistleblowing may be explored within a simulated scenario. All NHS organisations should now have a whistleblowers' policy, with transparent lines of responsibility to a senior management level. The GMC regards whistleblowing as a *professional responsibility*: 'You must protect patients when you believe that a doctor's or other colleague's health, conduct or performance is a threat to them'.[3]

The scenarios relating to Doctor Y above may be used as the basis for the simulation. Dr Y's behaviour deteriorates and Dr X has to inform someone about this. The group should discuss whom to inform and then run through the conversation with this person or body. The following alternative is a hospital-based scenario.

Learning outcomes

* The ethics of whistleblowing
* Dealing with a poorly performing colleague by talking to a senior colleague

For:

Hospital junior doctors including specialist registrars.

Location

Busy district general hospital.

Scenario

'Whistleblowing' participant (Doctor C)

'I am working as an SpR on a busy firm (specialty to reflect participant's own). I have been here for eight months. My boss Dr A is a wonderful clinician but I wouldn't really want to talk to him/her about personal matters. However I am concerned about Dr B, who is a junior consultant on my firm. I have watched her talking to patients and she is abrupt and often rude. She never interacts with the patients for long and certainly doesn't appear to discuss any concerns they may have about the treatment of their condition. The nurses have often asked me to talk to the patients after Dr B's ward round, and the patients often ask my opinion as "Dr B always seems so busy". Dr B often takes ages to answer her pager when she is the senior doctor on call above me. Yesterday one of her patients was crying and when I asked her why she said Dr B had told her that her condition was worsening and that soon there would be nothing that could be done for her. This may be the case but it doesn't seem the right way to tell a patient. I'm reluctant to but I think I will have to speak to Dr A about this. I am too scared to approach Dr B directly. The other registrars have told me to leave well alone as this could affect my reference, but I can't let the patients suffer and I am sure that Dr A will at least listen to my concerns.'

Simulated Doctor A

'Doctor C has asked to see me. He/she is a conscientious doctor who works very hard (sometimes too hard I think). I wonder what is wrong. My team are working well

---

Continued

> together. I have some good juniors. My fellow consultant, Dr B, who has been working here for one year in her first consultant post, is sometimes a bit brusque but she is an excellent clinician and clinically very skilled.'

Notes for facilitators

This scenario should be based as much as possible on the participants' own circumstances. Therefore it may stimulate some strong emotions. The scenario raises questions about professional behaviour and responsibility.

Interaction between a doctor and health professional

Learning outcome

* Ability to communicate with health professionals in difficult circumstances

For:

A mixed group of health professionals or students including doctors and pharmacists. A simulated professional is not needed for scenario 1 as participants may role-play the scenario after briefing.

Location

Either community or hospital.

Scenario 1

Dr E has prescribed a drug for patient MB but the dose is twice as high as that normally given to a woman of 75 years. The pharmacist rings Dr E to inform him/her of this.

Scenario 2

As above. Dr E is now played by the simulator. He/she is rather rude to the pharmacist and denies that the prescription is in any way at fault.

Scenario 3

As above. The pharmacist is now played by the simulator. He/she is rather rude to Dr E and tells him/her to be more careful in the future.

    These variations explore ways in which health professionals interact. A community pharmacist once told me that some GPs are quite rude when they are rung up about prescription errors. How should health professionals behave when a colleague is rude? This can lead to a discussion about telephone etiquette and responsibilities.

Summary

These scenarios reflect just a few of the types of interactions that occur between health professionals. They are good starting points for discussion.

References

1   British Medical Association. *Ethical responsibilities involved in treating doctor–patients.* London: British Medical Association, 1995.
2   *Oxford Dictionary of English* (2e). Oxford: Oxford University Press, 2003.
3   General Medical Council. *Duties of a Doctor: good medical practice.* London: General Medical Council, 1995.

Chapter 10

Formal interactions between professionals

This chapter explores:

- the appraisal process and how to prepare for it
- evaluation of posts
- disciplinary procedures
- supervisor–student interactions
- mentoring

The scenarios in this chapter prepare health professionals and students for the more formal interactions that occur during training and continuing professional development. In the same way that consultations between doctor and patient may be rehearsed and practised, so might appraisal interviewing, student support and the mentoring process, all of which are as important to the participants as the consultation is to doctor and patient.

Appraisals

Appraisals have become a fact of life for many health professionals. In the UK a GP must have an annual peer appraisal as a requirement to continue to practise. Appraisals are also taking place at undergraduate level with students undergoing appraisals at various times during their studies. Yet many appraisers have no formal training in giving this type of feedback, while appraisees are often understandably nervous of the process. A bad appraisal undermines confidence and is of no educational value.

Learning outcomes for sessions on appraisal

- To define the skills necessary for carrying out a successful appraisal
- To practise the skills in a non-threatening environment
- To develop strategies for dealing with more challenging appraisal scenarios
- To receive feedback on skills

Scenarios involving appraisals

If possible when running such sessions, the institution's official appraisal forms should be used in order to make the learning experience as authentic as possible. The participants for such workshops will be people learning to appraise, however all of them will probably also have experience of being appraised themselves. Before running the workshop it is useful to know how information is gathered before the interviews. What does the appraisee have to fill in? Are other members of staff asked for their opinions: e.g. 360 degree appraisal forms or peer review forms?

Problems often encountered by appraisers are: difficulty in giving 'negative' feedback or constructive criticism when there is cause for concern, this is particularly a problem if the appraisee has little or no insight; if the appraisee says little and is obviously anxious; if the appraiser concentrates only on the poorer part of performance and does not give feedback in relation to what the appraisee has done well or been successful in; when the appraisee has done extremely well and the appraiser gives praise without helping the appraisee to develop further.

The junior doctor

In this scenario the simulator is the junior doctor and one of the group members is the appraiser. The appraiser may wish to supply some details of his/her post in order to make the scenario more realistic (i.e. specialty, location etc).

Scenario for the simulated doctor

'I am Mark Davies halfway through my first pre-registration house officer post (three months of a six-month post). I am seeing Dr Wright for my mid-term appraisal. I enjoy medicine and do not feel that I have made any serious mistakes or caused staff any problems during my time on the wards. I was nervous at first and had some difficulties with basic skills such as putting in intravenous cannulae and taking blood gases. However these are no longer a problem as I have been putting myself in a position to do as many as possible. My knowledge base is good and I feel that I communicate well with patients and staff. I have found it hard to deal with the deaths of some of my elderly patients, particularly those I came to know well. I imagine I will get used to death in time. I do feel that there should be more day-to-day feedback given to me on the wards with regard to my performance, as often I have only my own self-assessment to go on.

I hope to tell my appraiser that there should be more regular feedback for junior doctors and not just criticism when we do something wrong. I would also like to talk about coping with death if my appraiser seems to have the time and asks me about any problems I am having.'

Information for the appraiser

Please note from the outset that there is no hidden agenda embedded in this scenario.

You have been asked to appraise Mark Davies as part of your normal duties as a specialist registrar/consultant in the department of general medicine at Wherever General Hospital.

Appraisee Mark Davies recently qualified from the University of Bigcity. Mark has been in your department for three months as part of a six-month placement as a pre-registration house officer (intern). Mark is a well-organised and keen intern still settling into this his first post. Your registrars and senior nurses are happy with Mark's performance on the wards. He interacts well with patients and often works late. His skills were not too good in his first few weeks but he is much better now and is an enthusiastic member of the team.

Notes for facilitators

There is little concern regarding Mark's performance but he is anxious to get some constructive feedback and would like to discuss how junior doctors adapt to coping with death. In the feedback session it is important that these issues are stressed by Mark if he has not had a chance to air them during the interview. The appraisal should be a two-way process and Mark should be given the time to discuss his needs. The group members also give feedback to the appraiser and discuss strategies for effective appraisals.

A junior doctor with some problems

Scenario for the simulated doctor

'I am Matthew Browne in my first post following my pre-registration (intern) year. I am now working in the emergency department at King's Cross Hospital. I am about to have my two-month appraisal with Dr Senior. I think that the appraisal will be fine. I get on well with all my colleagues and have a good laugh with the nurses in the department. I like to socialise after work and enjoy a few drinks, but am always on time for work and consider myself a true professional. My reports from my previous hospital, St Whatever were great and I did well at Bigtown University. I will be very surprised if there are any concerns raised during my appraisal.'

Information for the appraiser

You have been asked to appraise Matthew Browne two months after his start at King's Cross Hospital in the emergency department. This is his first year as a senior house officer (second foundation year). He has made quite an impression already; he is cheerful, confident and outgoing. He has demonstrated some good skills inserting intravenous lines and stitching. However department senior nurse (Selina Pread) has complained that Matthew is too familiar with the female nurses. He laughs and jokes with them and does not always present a professional demeanour in front of patients.

Appraisee Matthew Browne qualified from Bigtown University and has glowing reports for his intern positions at St Whatever Hospital.

Notes for facilitators

Matthew has a lack of insight into the effect his behaviour has in the department. Is the appraiser able to discuss this with him and enable him to see where the problem lies? The appraiser may not wish to delve too deeply into the issue, given that Matthew is otherwise doing well. What effect might this have in the long term?

Points for discussion

Ask participants what they think is the purpose of appraisal (*see* Box 10.1) and for their experiences of appraising and being appraised. Is the purpose likely to be perceived differently by appraiser and appraisee?

Box 10.1   Appraisal

Appraisal:
- is an official or formal evaluation of the strengths and weaknesses of someone (or something)
- should be a positive, formative and developmental process.

The purpose of appraisal
- To support staff
- To motivate
- To praise
- To improve quality: teaching, research, clinical standards
- May feed into revalidation

Brainstorm what should happen in an appraisal and compare this to what is expected at the institutions where participants work. Box 10.2 gives the appraisee's viewpoint and Box 10.3 the appraiser's.

Box 10.2   The appraisal process for the appraisee

The process: appraisee
- (Review last year's interview if appropriate)
- Collect information from day-to-day activities
- Refect on information collected
- Discuss and review information at appraisal
- Identify developmental and other needs

Information required
- Personal details
- Details of current activities: teaching, research, clinical
- Examples of good practice (student evaluation, grants, publications)
- Management activity
- Report on development action in last year
- Proposed objectives for next year

Areas to cover
- How good a teacher/clinician am I?
- How well do I perform?
- How do I measure my performance?
- How up to date am I?
- How well do I work in a team?
- What resources and support do I need?
- How well am I meeting my service objectives?
- What are my development needs?

Box 10.3   The appraisal process for the appraiser

The process: appraiser

- (Review last year and objectives)
- Discuss job performance and progress
- Praise!
- Identify development needs
- Discuss career plans
- Feedback
- Agree future action plan
- Possible fears/concerns of appraisee to consider
  - uncertainty about what the process will involve
  - lack of confidence in skills of appraiser
  - reluctance to reveal weaknesses in case penalised
- Time needed
- Possible lack of resources for professional development
- Possible lack of resources to remedy deficits
- Discuss how to improve performance
- Describe the problem in a friendly manner
- Point out specific behaviours
- Search and discuss the causes (skill, motivation, personal etc)
- Watch for avoidance
- Identify and write down solutions
- Decide on specific actions to take
- Agree on specific follow-up dates

Evaluation during a post: giving feedback on training

Junior doctors are often reluctant to give adverse feedback to their trainers about their training, due to concerns about future career prospects and references. Setting up a more formal evaluation interview during a post may help junior doctors feel more able to discuss their concerns. This scenario is similar to the one above where the hospital trainee gave feedback during appraisal. Here the trainer is not appraising the trainee but asking for his/her evaluation of the training process. The scenario takes place during general practice vocational training. This simulation is suitable for running at a half-day release session. The GP registrar may be able to develop the scenario from his or her own experience, or the following may be used.

Learning outcomes

- To give constructive feedback to more senior colleagues/trainers on their training and teaching
- To discuss strategies for dealing with training problems
- To explore barriers to feedback even if trainees have concerns

Scenario for the GP registrar

'I am Leslie Poole. I am four months into my three year GP vocational training programme and am working in a well-run practice of four partners and attached staff. My
workload is comfortable and I am able to attend the half-day release programme for
GP registrars at the local postgraduate centre every week. If ever I have a problem
dealing with a patient I am able to ask one of the doctors here for advice. This does
not happen too often. My main concern is that I am not getting the requisite number
of hours of formal tutorials each week. I should be sitting down with my trainer Dr S
for three hours during the week both to discuss set topics and to go through my cases.
I am lucky if we have one hour. Dr S is very busy with extra practice activities and is
always dashing off to meetings and clinics. If he over-runs his surgery in the morning
or has a lot of extra patients, the time for my training is eaten into and we often only
snatch half an hour or even less. However when we do manage to have the time, he is
a great teacher and mentor. I don't want to complain too much as I don't want to cause
any ill feelings between us, but I would like to talk about my patients with him, otherwise how will I ever learn?'

Scenario for the simulated trainer

' I have been a GP trainer for 10 years and love it. It is good to have a GP registrar in
the practice to take up some of the increasing workload, especially as I have so many
commitments at the moment. I do some occupational medicine and am on various committees. I am always willing to see extra patients at the end of surgery and don't mind
being interrupted by the GP registrar if she has a problem with a patient. I see this as
teaching time. Sometimes our more formal tutorials are a bit short, but overall I think
she gets a good deal: certainly better than I did when I was a registrar. None of my
registrars have ever complained about the practice and why should they? This is an
excellent place to learn. I have even introduced a time in the middle of the registrar's
training for her to give me feedback on my teaching skills. Excuse me I must dash,
I am 20 minutes late for the feedback session.'

Notes for facilitators

The interview should have a formal basis with the trainer or registrar setting out a formal agenda for discussion. In this way the two may be able to work through the issues,
as they know what is expected. The formal structure is one strategy of dealing with these
issues. The registrars may be able to think of others. Also explore how a registrar should
approach a trainer if there is no formal evaluation process.

Disciplinary procedures: an informal warning

This scenario involves a senior doctor asking to have an interview with a specialist registrar (SpR) outside the normal appraisal procedure because of concerns about the SpR's
work and attitude.

Scenario for the simulated registrar

'I am Robert Clarke. I have been working at this hospital as a specialist registrar for one year. I have good skills and a positive attitude to my work, which is up to date and has been praised by senior staff. I have shown a positive interest in training programmes for my specialty. Other staff have given me good appraisals in the past. I get on with patients and the nurses' and peers' 360 degree appraisal has been excellent. I usually dress smartly, look alert and professional and display a genuine sense of interest in those around me. I am a good team worker.'

Information for the senior doctor

Your task is to inform Robert that he is being informally warned that his behaviour is not acceptable. You will try to work with him to help him to change. You will try to find out the causes for his recent poor performance.

Robert does not know that recently colleagues on his team have commented on a change in his character. These comments have been from senior nursing staff and the more senior SpRs.

Dr E has noted an abruptness and lack of courtesy in Robert's reply when he asked Robert to cover him for two hours while he (Dr E) was appraised. This is usually something that colleagues do without question for each other.

Dr F noticed Robert leaving the ward 20 minutes or more early on several occasions and was surprised that Robert had not informed him before leaving the ward.

Dr G has made an informal complaint to the senior doctor that Robert left the ward without completing a patient history, which resulted in a delay in the patient having some investigation, causing some discomfort to the patient.

Dr H has had a row with Robert in earshot of patients. When Dr H asked Robert to cover an extra night duty Robert lost his temper and stormed off saying that he did all the work in this department. Dr H has also noticed Robert arriving late for duty in the morning on at least three occasions. He also remarks that Robert's shirt is not always well pressed.

Robert has also missed two sessions of his professional development programme.

Robert's personal information (for the simulated registrar)

You are married to Dianne Fox; she has moved to this town from a city 200 miles away in support of your medical career and has moved twice before. Dianne is starting her own business as a graphic designer and has now firmly asked you for reciprocal support in her career. You have a three-year-old child, Rebecca, who has asthma and eczema. Your neighbour looks after Rebecca when you are both at work. This neighbour, Mrs Monroe, does not like caring for Rebecca when the child is ill (has a cold, itchy skin, infected eczema). Under these circumstances Mrs Monroe phones Dianne and asks her to collect Rebecca. Recently Dianne has been phoning you to do this. Dianne has warned you that you owe her this support or the marriage is 'not worth it'. Dianne also starts work early some mornings, breakfast with clients, and you have to give Rebecca her food.

Now you have a difficult meeting with your senior doctor who has asked to see you this morning. You will not give anything away at this meeting. You just want to get through it without a formal warning; you believe you can fix things later.

If the doctor is forceful in finding out about the reasons for your poor performance you will say little and agree to an improvement even if you cannot see how you can manage it straight away. If challenged about time keeping you will say that you are doing more than your fair share of work. You always seem to be on night duty midweek (a time particularly difficult for you with Rebecca needing care). You think that you have covered the ward for more than your fair share of hours.

If asked about:

- the abrupt reply to Dr E you will say that there is no proper procedure for covering a temporary absence; you feel that *'I am asked too frequently'*
- Dr F noticing you leave early you will mention that staff *'never leave at the correct time'*. You often work late on other occasions
- Dr G complaining that you left the ward early and failed to clerk a patient fully, you will say that *'I thought I could have completed the details first thing in the morning with no problem to the patient'*. (You will be concerned that your own action has not been in the best interests of the patient.)
- rowing with Dr H when she requested an extra night duty from you, you will repeat your concern that: *'I am doing an unfair share of the rota . . . besides I should have been asked this question in private'* – you did not realise there were members of the public nearby
- failing to attend your own staff professional development session – you have missed two sessions now: *'I was too busy, I will catch up later'*.

Just how you respond to these allegations of professional misconduct depends on how the doctor talks to you. If questions are put in a non-judgemental and a balanced way you will listen and add your own perspective on the problem. You may give the interviewing doctor insight into difficult aspects of your problem, e.g. that Dianne has mentioned that she might leave you.

The more the interviewer gathers facts about the problem the more you may feel able to assist. You would be genuinely impressed and co-operative if you are offered options which may help with the situation. Can you feel any attempt at empathy with you? Then you would be likely to respond with your own evaluation and ideas to improve. If you cannot see a positive way out say so unless the doctor is, in your opinion, not interested. You may suggest that you both monitor the situation.

Points for discussion

Here are some good options a good interviewer is likely to bring out in the interview:

- child minding facilities at the hospital for Rebecca
- examining the rota with an independent person to verify that you are not working an unfair share of hours and that the rota is not unbalanced
- checking the possibility that you could arrange to work at a time that suits your needs e.g. so you can pick up Rebecca from the crèche at 4:30 pm but you pay the time back by agreement with your colleagues
- would you be prepared to apologise to certain staff?
- would you like the doctor to inform staff – discreetly – of your current difficulty?

The mark of a good interviewer is the degree to which Robert feels involved in solving the problem.

Supervision of student projects/postgraduate degrees

Health professionals are often involved in the supervision of students' research projects, junior doctors' audits and qualified professionals' undertaking higher certificates, diplomas and masters degrees. The supervisor–student relationship is another interaction that may be simulated. Supervisors may receive training in supervision but this is usually theoretical rather than experiential. Likewise students are rarely trained in how to get the best from their supervision.

Learning outcomes

- Discussion of the nature of the student–supervisor relationship
- Communication strategies for student–supervisor interactions
- Getting the best from supervision

This simulation involves a student interacting with his/her supervisor. Either the student or the supervisor may be played by a simulator, or both roles may be played by group participants depending on the focus of the session. The level of the student is decided depending on the group with whom the facilitator is working. For example if the group is made up of GP trainers, then this may be a simulated registrar, who is receiving advice about a project from the GP. Or this may be a simulated doctor undertaking a masters degree who has a supervisor for his/her dissertation. If the session involves a mixed group of students and supervisors, then the facilitator may introduce a simulated supervisor, or ask both roles to be played by group members. Following the 'scripted' scenario below, the facilitator may ask group participants to describe any problems they have had/are having with supervision, so that these may be 'acted out' and discussed.

Information for the student

You are at an early stage in your project/degree. You will be discussing your literature review and how it leads into your research questions with your supervisor for the fourth time! During past interactions with him/her you have been asked to change the way you present the literature review, to add more references and to be more logical in how your research questions derive from gaps in the current literature. This is the first time you have had to write an academic-type paper since qualification, and you are a bit rusty about literature searches. Now:

- you are very pleased with it
- you are particularly confident that your research questions are 'big'
- you have put in a lot of time and effort – nearly three months every night in the library after work to read, write, rewrite and edit
- in your opinion your literature review is looking very impressive and you feel confident that this will impress your supervisor as it has your peers.

This time you are sure your supervisor will be pleased. If, however, the supervisor is still not satisfied, you will feel very frustrated and try to argue your case. You will say that other people who have read it have been very complimentary and feel you have done an excellent job. You want to understand exactly what the problem is but feel that your supervisor is not in touch with your ideas.

Information for supervisor

You have been supervising Sam for four months. He/she has been working on a literature review for a research project. You feel that despite the number of drafts and the time spent on the work it is still not right. You expect more relevant and up-to-date references and a more logical lead-in to the research question. You do not understand why Sam is having such a problem with the project. He/she is obviously not spending enough time on it.

Points for discussion

It is quite difficult to role-play the above scenario without a real literature review or project. However it may be used as a starting point for discussion about the role of a supervisor, the student–supervisor 'formal' interactions, and how to give constructive guidance about written work.

Mentoring

Health professionals, whether clinical, academic or both, are likely to enter into a mentoring role with a junior colleague or student during their careers. They may be a mentor in an official capacity or unofficially. One definition of mentoring is:

> *'A process whereby an experienced, highly regarded, empathic person (the mentor), guides another individual (the mentee) in the development and re-examination of their own ideas, learning, and personal and professional development. The mentor . . . achieves this by listening and talking in confidence to the mentee'.*[1]

As is the case with supervision, often there is no formal training for mentoring. The communication skills required are, of course, similar to those used in doctor–patient consultations, appraisals and one-to-one teaching. When running a group session for potential and ongoing mentors, the scenarios developed to role-play with a simulated mentee should be based on participants' experience of the mentoring process and any problems they may have encountered with mentees. The encounters may then be re-rehearsed and re-run for future interactions. (*See* Chapter 11 for developing on-the-spot scenarios.) In particular, mentors may wish to work through scenarios involving conflict of some kind.

Handling conflict within professional interactions

Conflict may occur during any human interaction. The scenarios in this chapter involve various levels of conflict. Once a scenario has been worked through, participants in the learning group should be able to devise their own tips for dealing with conflict. These will probably be similar to those in Box 10.4 (drawn from the further reading list at the end of the chapter).

Box 10.4   Resolving conflict

- Ensure that the meeting takes place in a comfortable, and preferably, neutral environment.

Continued

- Set a time limit for the interaction.
- Both parties should acknowledge that conflict exists.
- Establish rules for the interaction during which the conflict is to be resolved, i.e. no raising voices, listen, do not interrupt.
- Explore why the conflict has arisen and what may be learnt from this to avoid conflict in the future.
- Consider the options for resolving the conflict, e.g. compromise, collaboration, co-operation.
- Face up to cultural differences if these are implicated in the conflict.
- Try to understand both points of view.
- Attempt to resolve the conflict by negotiation, as unresolved conflict will ultimately affect the relationship.
- Look at all sides of the argument, suspending judgement until this is done.
- Devise an action plan for further interactions and resolution.
- If necessary invite a conciliator to the interaction to facilitate.

Summary

Appraisals, disciplinary interviews and mentoring are common tasks that health professionals face, often with little training. Rehearsing the skills through simulations helps with the real processes and should make participants more comfortable in these situations.

Reference

1 Standing Committee on Postgraduate Medical and Dental Education (SCOPME). *Supporting Doctors and Dentists at Work. An enquiry into mentoring.* London: SCOPME, 1998.

Further reading

- Bayley H, Chambers R and Donovan C. *The Good Mentoring Toolkit for Healthcare.* Oxford: Radcliffe Medical Press, 2004.
- Chambers R, Tavahie A, Mohanna K and Wakley G. *The Good Appraisal Toolkit for Primary Care.* Oxford: Radcliffe Medical Press, 2004.
- Chambers R, Wakley G, Field S and Ellis S. *Appraisal for the Apprehensive: a guide for doctors.* Oxford: Radcliffe Medical Press, 2003.
- Elwyn G, Greenhalgh T and Macfarlane F. *Groups. A guide to small group work in healthcare, management and research.* Oxford: Radcliffe Medical Press, 2001.

Chapter 11

Developing scenarios in response to students' and professionals' needs

> This chapter explores:
> - the learning needs of participants
> - developing scenarios to meet those needs.

Pre-scripted scenarios are useful in many types of learning sessions and help save time, as new scenarios do not need to be written. However, for more senior students and experienced clinicians, to maximise the learning potential it is possible to develop roles and scenarios before or during sessions in response to learning needs. Junior students tend to focus on what communication skills they need to pass an examination. As they have very little clinical experience, if any, such students find it difficult to suggest scenarios upon which to base a learning session. Scenario development may also be difficult with learners new to simulated patient work.

Senior students and clinicians are able to suggest scenarios stimulated by the difficulties they face in their everyday interactions. Experienced consultants with years of clinical work behind them may suggest very specific scenarios and, through working through these, develop strategies and gain feedback on how to improve their communication skills.

In the early years of communication skills development, scenarios are chosen by the course organisers to meet outcomes defined in the curriculum. In communication workshops we do not necessarily want the agenda to be restricted to such topics as breaking bad news, even though this is often the one for which learners ask. There are many other intricate situations that clinicians face that are suitable for working through in partnership with SPs.

Ways in which scenarios may be generated

In the planning stages of a workshop

When developing ideas for workshops we start by looking at the participants with whom we will be working. There may be a well-defined topic for the sessions. However if there are flexible learning outcomes, and it is possible to contact the participants beforehand, the scenarios may be developed from the real-life encounters of the participants. Organisers can send out a pre-course questionnaire and ask for scenario ideas or areas of difficulty that the participants wish to work through. What are *their* learning needs?

For example a group of interprofessional educators at Leeds Medical School developed a set of workshops for pre-registration house officers, pre-registration pharmacists and final year nursing students, to facilitate interprofessional working following qualification. A few weeks before the workshops we asked the three groups to write down any situations they had encountered in which there had been problems or difficulties in working with their colleagues from another health profession. We used some of the responses to develop three scenarios to work through in the subsequent workshops.[1,2]

The scenarios written by the learner in advance of the learning session are often short on detail. A skilled facilitator will be able to identify what it is the learner wants to experience and, with the SP, can develop a simulation from an outline. The subsequent story depends to a degree on the availability of suitable SPs: sex, age and ability to perform the role.

On the day

Participants may be asked to provide details of difficulties, in the first stages of a workshop. This is best done once the learning group has formed and the learners are comfortable in discussing what might be quite sensitive topics. Admitting difficulties of communication or interactions with patients may be daunting for less experienced learners. Admitting difficulties with staff either junior or senior may be even more so. A prepared SP role may be useful to help break the ice.

Topics that are often suggested in such sessions are shown in Box 11.1.

Box 11.1   Examples of participant-generated scenarios

- Eliciting a menstrual history
- Eliciting a sexual history
- How to deal with a patient who starts crying
- How to deal with an aggressive patient
- Dealing with a patient who unexpectedly volunteers she has been the victim of domestic violence or sexual abuse
- When a relative asks for information about a patient
- When a relative says that a patient should not be told a poor prognosis
- Dealing with a poorly performing receptionist
- Disciplining another health professional
- Interviewing a poorly performing medical student
- Tackling a colleague suspected of alcohol or drug abuse
- Tactfully dealing with a colleague who seeks a corridor consultation
- Admitting a medical mistake
- Appearing in court
- Appearing at an inquiry

Developing scenarios from patients

Working with patient groups is a useful way of developing scenarios; patients often talk about communication difficulties with their healthcare providers. SPs are also 'real' patients, and may also be asked to give examples that they think are worthy of working up into roles. However it is not best practice to ask SPs to 'play' themselves. This needs careful discussion between the facilitator and SP.

Developing scenarios on the day

Obviously if participants suggest topics prior to the learning session, it is easier to prepare SPs and any support material. For SPs to develop roles on the day, we need to have a highly trained group of SPs who are able to adapt and feel their way into unfamiliar roles with empathy and insight.

As participants could volunteer all sorts of encounters and there will always be surprises, facilitators should be watchful that SPs do not become anxious or upset by scenarios that may bring back memories of events in their past. The SPs may not have time to discuss their reluctance to take on a particular role, for example a woman who is the victim of domestic violence. An SP may have been in this situation herself.

Box 11.2 lists some ways in which scenarios may be generated on the day.

Box 11.2   How to generate ideas

- Ask students to think about skills that they need on the wards or in the community: what worries them about interacting with patients?
- What skills do students wish to practise before an examination (e.g. ability to finish off an interview)?
- Ask participants to think about an incident they have seen on a ward round: something positive that they wish to practise; something negative they wish to work through.
- What critical incidents have happened recently (e.g. having to break bad news and feeling unprepared; an incident in which a patient or relative became aggressive)?
- Some students may want to know how to set boundaries: dealing with a flirtatious or overfamiliar patient.
- Ask participants to describe something they have seen on TV or read about in a newspaper that they wish to enact because they weren't sure how they would have dealt with the situation.
- Registrars might want to practise appraisals; consultants might want to rehearse interactions with hospital management.
- What problems have arisen recently in relation to interprofessional communication and relationships? Healthcare teams are complex.
- Trainers may recently have had to deal with difficult students/registrars in groups.

Advice for facilitators

Even if the aim of the session is to work through scenarios generated by the group, it is usually a good idea for the facilitator to have three or four *pre-scripted* scenarios. This helps the group in several ways. The *pre-written* scenarios allow students to warm up and naturally start discussing the experiential learning techniques. It takes the pressure off the facilitator by not depending on the group to generate ideas they want to develop early in the session. While using a pre-scripted role the facilitator may also reaffirm the safe learning environment: that it is all right to make mistakes during role-play, as these can be discussed and worked through again. On the day the facilitator and the students may be meeting for the first time, working through one *ready-written* role brings the group together, and reminds them of the ways to give feedback. The facilitator should mention at the beginning of the exercise that the true purpose of the session is to work through roles and situations that the learners are most interested in, that have meaning for them and that would help them with their current attachments.

These sessions, in which roles are generated on the day, are much tougher for the facilitator than just working through pre-scripted scenarios. The facilitator has to have an already established rapport or be able to establish one quickly if the group is new. For the latter case the first pre-scripted scenario is also a good rapport builder.

Let's move on now to generating a role that *belongs* to the students to be used within an hour's session. How is this done?

It is possible that the pre-session briefing included instructions to the participants to be prepared to share experiences that they wish to work through in the group. The briefing can include the various starting points as listed in Box 11.2. In group learning sessions the facilitator may have access to say five simulators. These simulators should be experienced rather than novices. Each simulator usually has five or six roles of which he or she is very confident. The simulators represent a pool of 30 types of learner/simulator interactions albeit with some overlap in roles. A learner wants to experience how to talk to a patient who is very emotional. The facilitator can ask the group of SPs who wants to deliver that role and usually obtain a match. If a role is requested and no SP is experienced in it, then the SPs will help decide who is best for the role and possibly give advice on how it might be played.

Viewpoint of a simulated patient

When I know that I will be involved in playing a role the nature of which will be developed during the learning session I take a change of clothes. I prefer to dress in a smart dark suit, white shirt and collar and tie at the beginning. It is much easier to dress down with the aid of a few props: trainers, tee shirt, track suit bottoms and the dreaded base ball cap, than to smarten up! I wear my hair very short so that I might pass myself off as sporty aggressive or merely balding.

In my opinion it is easy to play an aggressive patient who will get more and more out of control if the interviewer allows. I have witnessed real patients behave like this, both male and female, and my character is a composite. This is almost like playing to the gallery. So if a facilitator asks who wants to play an aggressive patient, I do. For this role it does not matter how I dress. I sit/stand too close to the interviewer, raise my voice or even lower it and make my demands. Whether I am suited or track-suited I usually get what I want, which may not be what I need. This role affords the following learning points for the interviewer:

- meeting and greeting the patient firmly
- maintaining eye contact and respectful language
- never threatening the patient
- negotiating with the patient rather than refusing a need (quicker treatment, more time/drugs or acknowledging a mistake)
- terminating a damaging interview.

If a group participant wants me to re-enact a very specific incident and recreate the problem or challenge that the learner wants to improve on, I need to know the designation of the person to be simulated (patient, doctor, health professional, relative etc).

Working with students

Students are often tired and emotional, stressed, scared and reluctant to volunteer ideas to generate scenarios. No-one wants to be first in the hot seat. Students do not want to be judged, they want to appear as if they are in control in front of their peers. The facilitator has to stress that they are not being assessed and that this is an opportunity for them to rehearse difficult situations in a safe and non-threatening environment, and to receive feedback.

Summary

Generating scenarios 'on the day' is a skilful process and requires experienced facilitators and simulated patients.

References

1   Kilminster SM, Stark P, Hale C *et al*. Can interprofessional education workshops affect interprofessional communication? *J Interprof Care*. 2003; **17**: 199–200.
2   Kilminster SM, Stark P, Hale C *et al*. Learning for real life: patient focussed interprofessional workshops do offer added value. *Med Educ*. 2004; **38**: 717–26.

Chapter 12

Simulated patients and assessment

This chapter explores:

- assessing competence and performance in relation to communication and consultation skills
- designing an assessment: validity and reliability
- methods of assessment
- assessment scales
- standard setting
- assessment by simulated patients and observers
- quality assurance
- formative and summative assessment
- examples of scenarios for assessment.

Assessment of communication and consultation skills may be carried out by a variety of methods. There are trends in assessment just as there are trends in other aspects of clinical education. The method of assessment will depend on the level of the examination: high stakes such as medical finals or professional examinations, or university end of year examinations for example. Because of the underlying topic of this book we will only consider assessment in relation to the use of SPs.

Competence and performance

The first thing to consider when developing an assessment is the difference between competence and performance (*see* definitions in Box 12.1). Each assessment method may be used for one or the other.

Box 12.1   Some definitions

Competence: the ability to do the job. What doctors do in controlled representations of professional practice.[1] *Assessment by OSCE; observed simulated consultations.*

Performance: the ability to do the job well. What doctors do in their professional practice.[1] *Assessment by incognito simulated patients.*

Competence relates to the 'shows how' of Miller's pyramid, and performance to the 'does' (*see* Box 12.2). A health professional may demonstrate competence in an examination but may perform poorly at times in the clinical setting. In most consultation skills examinations we are assessing competence.

Box 12.2 Miller's pyramid[2]

- Assessment of 'knows' by written examinations such as multiple choice questions or oral examinations
- Assessment of 'knows how' by written examinations that test diagnostic reasoning such as matching pairs or modified essay questions, plus orals
- Assessment of 'shows how' by clinical examinations: *competence*
- Assessment of 'does' in the workplace with real *performance*

Designing an assessment

There are a series of questions to be answered when designing an assessment of communication/consultation skills (*see* Box 12.3). Validity and reliability are particularly important for high stakes examinations (*see* Box 12.4). However, validity is often gained at the expense of reliability and vice versa. Inter-case reliability is perhaps the most important issue in communication skills testing, as students, qualified professionals and examinees do not perform consistently from consultation to consultation.[3] Moreover, one study has shown that doctors do not perform the same way with the same patient with the same story consulting six weeks apart (intra-doctor variation).[4] To make a valid judgement of a person's communication and/or consultation competence, a large number of scenarios involving a broad variety of clinical presentations and patients need to be observed and assessed. This is not so crucial in the early years of training, and indeed is not feasible given the number of students in each year of undergraduate training. However for finals and professional examination the number of cases is important.

Box 12.3 Designing a communication skills assessment

---

1 What is the purpose of the assessment?
2 Who is to be tested?
3 What aspects of competence or performance are to be measured?
4 What method(s) should be used?
5 How are the scores to be defined?
6 What is the reliability of the assessment?
7 Is the assessment valid?
8 What are the standards against which the candidates are to be measured?

Box 12.4 Validity and reliability

Validity
How well a test or instrument measures what it should be measuring.
We would hope to be able to say: 'The higher the score, the better an examinee's communication/consultation skills'.

Continued

> **Reliability**
> The reproducibility or consistency of a test.
>
> - *Inter-rater reliability*: the ability of a test or instrument to produce similar results/scores when used by different observers: 'An examinee's score for an assessment should be similar when marked by two or more observers at the same time'.
> - *Intra-rater reliability*: the ability of a test or instrument to produce similar results/scores when used by the same observer on different days: 'An examinee should be scored the same if marked on different days by the same person'.
> - *Inter-case (candidate) reliability*: the ability of a test to measure consistency of an examinee's performance across cases. An examinee's marks should be broadly similar for each consultation in a series of such cases.

Methods of assessment

Assessing 'shows how' with simulated patients

These assessments are for end-point examinations in which the examinees should be able to demonstrate they have reached an appropriate level of competence at their stage of training. Such a demonstration means they are able to move on to the next level. Failure should result in some form of remediation. What competencies are being examined should be defined, and the marking sheet should reflect this.

There are a number of methods that may be used. For junior students one or two SP interactions may be sufficient, in combination with a group facilitator's comments on a student's skills during training sessions. For senior students, particularly for 'finals' and for postregistration assessments, more interactions are needed across an examination blueprint. (The blueprint is a map of the whole assessment procedure to ensure that the candidate is being examined across all competencies.) This should also be combined with feedback about a candidate's performance in the clinical setting from a variety of sources including peers, patients and other professionals (i.e. multisource feedback, 360 degree appraisal).

The OSCE

A common format for the assessment of communication skills within a broader clinical skills examination (also assessing physical examination and procedural skills) is the OSCE (objective structured clinical examination). Developed by Harden and Gleeson in 1979, the OSCE is now commonplace at medical schools and for some professional examinations.[5] The OSCE consists of a number of stations that help to give adequate sampling across various clinical scenarios and skills. Candidates rotate through the stations, which typically last from five to 15 minutes. There may be stations designated as specific 'communication' skills stations, or the majority of stations may include some elements of communication. For example there may be one station for information gathering (an SP with a complicated history) and one for information giving (explanation of a procedure to an SP). At other stations, such as examining the abdomen, candidates may receive marks for 'introducing oneself', 'explaining the examination to the patient' and 'being courteous'.

The OSCE is certainly a useful tool; however it is limited by the length of the stations. Thus skills are often broken down into components such as information gathering, examination of one body system or one clinical procedure. Some OSCEs we have observed may even include 'breaking bad news' or discussing an unwanted pregnancy (the latter was a five-minute station at one medical school). While it is possible to have a long (or double station) we would question the wisdom of having only eight or even 16 minutes for such complex tasks. Brevity gives a wrong message to students in particular. While the standard length of a British consultation in general practice may be just under ten minutes (9.36 minutes in 1997;[6] 9.4 minutes in 2004[7]), assessment of the complexity of the skills involved in difficult patient interactions should reflect what we would want to happen in such situations. Moreover, doctor–patient interactions in many consultations are rarely one-off situations, and real-life consultations may be shorter because the patient's background is already familiar to the clinician.

OSCEs require a deep pool of well-trained SPs, some of whom are prepared to be examined if real patients with physical signs are not involved. As with all these assessments, consistency is vital to ensure reliability. The SP must react in the same way to the same question and/or stimulus.

Assessment of communication skills in an OSCE can be difficult as some skills are case-specific.[3] Excellent communication with one patient may be followed by poor communication with another, particularly if the candidate is stressed by a patient's condition about which he/she has minimal knowledge. Also examinees may do well on a checklist of items, for example asking about a patient's concerns, without fully understanding or engaging with the process.[8] An examinee's level of competence is not generalisable across stations. To assess empathy, for example, as many as 37 different cases would be needed.[9] However by collating the communication aspects of all stations in one examination there is a reasonable assessment of a candidate's skills.

The simulated surgery

While the OSCE has its advantages and perhaps mirrors to some extent the behaviour of professionals in certain situations such as working on wards (going from bed to bed) or in the emergency department, the outpatient or general practice way of consulting is not simulated. To improve authenticity we can use the simulated surgery method. Introduced in 1997 the simulated surgery allows assessment of such consultation skills as problem solving, clinical management, personal care, oral communication and the totality of the consultation process. Physical examination skills are usually not tested.[10]

The usual format of the surgery involves eight to 12 cases lasting up to ten minutes each. The examinee sits in the 'consulting room' and the SPs rotate round the rooms.

Assessing 'does' by clinical examinations

Ultimately the most valid assessment of consultation and communication skills and clinical performance is by testing what a health professional does in the workplace: in hospital and in the general practice surgery. This is an assessment of 'does', the professional's actual performance, and is restricted to assessments after initial qualification. The only assessment of 'does' involving SPs is by the use of incognito SPs.

Incognito simulated patients

Also known as covert SPs in contrast with overt, this method has not been used extensively in the UK.[11] However in the Netherlands, SPs have been involved in posing as 'real' patients for the assessment of GPs' performance and also in secondary care settings.[12,13]

The use of SPs in this way has been shown to be a valid method for assessing actual clinical performance in the workplace.[14]

The rationale is that if the doctors are unaware that the patient is an SP, their clinical performance is likely to be more authentic. However there are logistical problems to overcome when trying to introduce an SP into a general practice surgery or other setting without the doctor knowing.[15] This limits the feasibility of the method. Moreover this method does raise ethical issues.[16]

Marking sheets

With any of these methods a marking sheet or scale is required. In the early years of training these are often devised just before the examination and are not subject to validation or tests of reliability in any formal sense. They are usually specific to the scenario (*see* examples below). Alternatively a validated instrument may be used. These include more generalised items and may need to be adapted for a particular scenario. The scale may be completed by the SP, a medically trained observer or assessor (usually senior to the candidate), a peer for revalidation purposes, or a combination of these. Rating scales vary not only in content but also in the method of marking. Some have Likert scales, some have defined parameters, and some have space to write in comments, while others grade simply as pass/fail.

There are a large number of scales and assessment instruments available for assessing communication/consultation skills. Those that are published have usually been evaluated for validity and reliability to some extent. Some scales focus on content and some on process. Some try to combine both elements. Detailed checklists have been shown not to be as objective as originally thought.[17] Global marking, that is when an examiner gives a single mark based on his/her opinion of the candidate's skills, has been shown to be as reliable as long as the examiners receive adequate training.[18] However checklists are useful for giving candidates feedback, if this is built into the assessment procedure, or for providing proof of what happened in the assessment if a candidate contests his/her marks. Checklists also drive behaviour, as they show examinees what is expected of them. It is beyond the scope of this book to go into these in any detail.

Setting standards or the 'pass mark'

A pass mark must be set at the most fitting level for the level of expertise expected of the examinees. Standard setting is usually done by criterion referencing and is decided before the assessment is marked. This is in contrast to peer referencing in which passing or failing is described relative to the position of other candidates and when only a preset number of candidates are allowed to pass the assessment. When carried out to the highest degree of accuracy, criterion referencing should involve setting standards for each element of an assessment, item by item. Thus it is not sufficient to set a pass mark of 50% for each station or the whole of an examination. There are a number of methods of setting standards, and there are references for interested readers at the end of the chapter. Probably the most commonly used for OSCEs is the modified Angoff procedure. The original method described by Angoff in 1971 involved a panel of experts independently estimating how a hypothetical candidate with borderline competence would perform on each of the test items.[19] The modified method is a simpler procedure that allows for discussion and consensus, but is still time-consuming to do properly. For early assessments the pass mark will be set without detailed mathematical discussion.

Assessment by simulated patients

When assessing communication skills by any method, the assessor may be an observer and/or the SP. SPs are able to give feedback in training sessions. Assessment is thus an extension of this role. The evidence suggests that SPs can assess examinees' competence reliably.[20] Only patients can really say if they have understood what the doctor has told them, if they felt involved in decision making and if their views were valued. However SPs cannot assess medical knowledge: they may be provided with checklists written by professionals to help them to do this. For example when running a simulated surgery, the method is more lifelike if there is no extra observer in the consulting room. The SP is in charge of marking and has two sheets for the assessment. The first clinical sheet is a series of items that are specific to the case, for example if a patient complains of cough the candidate would be marked on whether he or she asked about family history. The clinical sheet is objective in that the SP does not know the relative weighting of each item and is only marking on the basis of what the doctor says or does. The communication sheet is more subjective and is based on what the patient (in role) feels about the doctor's skills in relation to rapport building, explaining skills and involving the patient in management decisions. Examples of scoring on this sheet are: 'I understood what the doctor told me'; 'I felt comfortable with this doctor'; 'I would consult this doctor again'.

Quality assurance of assessments

During high stakes examinations there are usually 'floating' assessors who visit each station of an OSCE to ensure that the examination protocol is being followed. This allows for monitoring of SP performance to ensure consistency of the role with each candidate, and double marking of some candidates to check reliability. The QA examiner may also comment on the suitability of roles in action and whether they need modification if used again.

Formative and summative assessment

SPs may be asked to give both formative and summative assessment as discussed above. The ideal summative assessment should include feedback and so it is also formative. However after most end-point assessments, the only feedback the examinees receive is in the form of whether they have passed or failed. There may be a mark or grade. If possible, when planning assessments in the early years of medical and health professional training, build in time for feedback. Thus after a ten-minute communication skills assessment at the end of first year of medical school, add an extra five minutes for feedback from observer and/or SP. Otherwise the educational nature of the experience is lost. Of course an extra five minutes per candidate is time-consuming if the year group is over 200. But just giving students their marking sheets back later is not going to be of great use: feedback is more successful if timely and immediate.

Examples of scenarios used for assessments

Many of the scenarios given in earlier chapters may be adapted for use in assessment. A marking sheet will be needed and standard setting should be carried out.

First year medical students: basic communication/interviewing skills: gathering information

Competencies being assessed

* Introduction
* Verbal and non-verbal communication skills
* Patient-centred approach: exploration of ideas, concerns and expectations
* Summarising

Patient's name

Sam Cowan, age about 50 years (patient may be male or female).
Assessed by an observer with input from the SP.

Information for candidates

You will have a maximum of *8 minutes* in which to demonstrate your ability to interact with a patient as a medical student interviewing the patient before he/she sees the GP. A timer will be started immediately you enter the examination room. *When the buzzer sounds at 8 minutes you must finish the interview.* (If used as a formative assessment the observer may then give feedback for three minutes.)

Instructions to the student

1   Read the scenario and be prepared to interview the patient.
2   Towards the end of the interview you should summarise your 'history' and give the patient an indication of what you perceive his/her problems to be.
3   The facilitator will assess you on a structured mark sheet (and at the end of the interview give you feedback on your communication skills).
4   Below is some prior information for you to consider before entering the room.

Scenario

Sam Cowan is a 50-year-old estate agent. He/she has made an appointment to see the GP in the local practice. You ask if you can interview him/her before going in to see the doctor.

Information for the simulated patient

When asked why you have come to see the doctor today you will reply:

> *'I've been finding it difficult to concentrate at work recently and I was wondering if my blood pressure was up again.'*

You are a 50-year-old estate agent. For the past month you have been finding it difficult to concentrate at work and interact with your clients. You used to enjoy the whole of your job especially when you were able to clinch a sale. You are good at what you do and have been successful so far. You have no money worries.

Two years ago you were diagnosed with high blood pressure (hypertension) and take one tablet a day for this (a beta-blocker). Your blood pressure has been well controlled for the last 18 months and your medication has not been changed in that time. Though you are aware that the tablets can make you feel tired, you do not think it likely that these are causing your symptoms as you have been on them so long. However you would like the doctor to check your blood pressure today in case it has gone up.

You are happily married. Your spouse works for the local town council. You have two daughters aged 20 and 16 years.

If specifically asked

- About sleep: you find it more difficult to get off to sleep at the moment. You lie awake for about an hour, but once you are asleep you sleep through the night and get up OK in the morning.
- You do not smoke.
- You drink about four units at the weekend, rarely during the week (either beer or wine).
- You watch what you eat and try to do some exercise like walking most days but sometimes this is difficult as you often work long hours. Your appetite has not changed.

If asked about your ideas about the problem

You wonder if the lack of concentration is related to blood pressure and this is certainly what you would like checking first.

If asked about any worries

You are reluctant at first to mention this but you have been worried about your older daughter who is 20 and studying geography at the local university. She is in second year. She did very well in her exams and assignments in year 1 but this year you have noticed that she doesn't seem to be studying as much. She lives at home and is often out till after midnight most nights, and at the weekends she rarely gets home before morning. She tells you that she is studying at uni, but you are not sure that this is the case. She seems irritable and has lost weight. You are worried that she might be taking drugs. You don't know much about this but you are aware that a lot of young people smoke cannabis or take Ecstasy if they go out to clubs. You have tried to talk to her about this but she gets annoyed and goes to her room. Your spouse is not concerned and does not want to get involved in an argument: anything for a quiet life. You do not think this is really a problem for the doctor but it will probably help to talk it over with someone else. You do not expect any easy answers about what to do, but some leaflets on drugs may be useful.

If asked you will probably agree that this worry may be causing your lack of concentration.

Your other daughter is fine.

If asked what you hope the doctor will be able to do to help you

- First you hope he will check your blood pressure.
- If you have mentioned your daughter, you would like the doctor to listen to your concerns and perhaps give you some information about drugs.

You are otherwise fit and well. (If female your periods are still regular and you do not think you are on the change.)

Marking

The clinical observer gives the mark out of 20. The SP gives a mark out of 5. Tables 12.1 and 12.2 give examples of mark sheets for this scenario. Possible totals are shown in bold in Table 12.1.

Table 12.1 Mark sheet: completed by clinical observer

Competency/behaviour	Mark
1 Introduces self and asks for reason for visit	0
	1
2 Uses appropriate body language throughout interview:	
Eye contact	1
Body posture (relaxed but attentive)	1
Shows warmth to patient	1
	3
3 Voice projection (audible, not shy or embarrassed)	0
	1
4 Uses appropriate question style throughout consultation:	
Open questions used effectively	1
Closed questions used effectively	1
Encouragers used when appropriate	1
	3
5 Uses appropriate question technique:	
Empathic	1
Focuses on patient rather than on the physical complaint alone	1
	2
6 History taking:	
History of hypertension	1
On treatment: not changed	1
Lifestyle (sleep, appetite etc)	1
	3
7 Identifies patient's ideas and concerns:	
BP up and would like it measured	1
Concern about daughter	2
Would like some information on drugs	2
	5
8 Closes the interview:	
Summarises	1
Asks if patient has anything else to add	1
	2
Mark	**/20**

Table 12.2 Global performance: marked by simulated patient

Poor: didn't put you at ease, poor listening skills, didn't explore your concerns		Satisfactory: put you at ease, listened well, explored your concerns, missed some of the history		Excellent: put at ease, student empathic, felt able to discuss all concerns, all essential elements of your history covered	
0	1	2	3	4	5

Final year medical students: consultation involving initial management of diabetes including information giving and patient-centred approach

This consultation requires about 16 minutes and would probably be a double station in most OSCEs.

Competencies being assessed

- Diagnosis of type 2 diabetes
- Communication skills, in particular sharing/giving information with minimal jargon
- Adopting a patient-centred approach with exploration of the patient's concerns
- Ability to check patient's understanding
- Applied knowledge of type 2 diabetes so information given to the patient is correct

Instructions to the student

You have *16 minutes* to perform the tasks listed.

Scenario

You are a pre-registration house officer (intern) working in general practice. Mark Johnson, aged 56 years, is returning to see you in your general practice for the results of some investigations. He presented to the surgery last week and saw a locum doctor.

Medical notes from 1 week ago
Three-month history of lethargy and one month of urinary frequency. No dysuria. Nocturia × 2 per night. Weight loss: thinks about 3 kg in last month. Non-smoker. Twenty units of alcohol per week (beer). Works for council: park maintenance. Married with two children.

Past medical history
Appendicectomy age 22 years.

Family history
Father died age 75 years: myocardial infarction.
Mother age 80 years alive and well.
Maternal grandmother: diabetes.

Examination
BP 138/84 mmHg, BMI 30. Otherwise unremarkable (CVS (cardiovascular system), RS (respiratory system) and abdomen).

Investigations
FBE [full blood examination], U&Es [urea and electrolytes], LFTs [liver function tests], TFTs [thyroid function tests]: all normal.
Fasting blood sugar: 12.5 mmol/l
Fasting cholesterol: 6.2 mmol/l
Urine test: glucose ++, no protein, no growth, no ketones

Tasks for students

You are required to:
1 Discuss these results with Mr Johnson.
2 Advise him of the diagnosis.
3 Agree on a management plan.

NB: You do *not* need to examine him in this consultation.

Information for the simulated patient

You are Mark Johnson, aged 56 years. You came to the surgery/general practice last week and saw a locum doctor. You have not met the doctor you are seeing today before. You have been feeling tired for about three months. You are not sure why. Your job is physically demanding but you have had no trouble before. You are sleeping well. You have also noticed that you have been going to the toilet to pass urine more often in about the last month. You get up twice in the night to urinate (prior to the last few weeks you would occasionally get up once). There has been no burning or stinging and you have a good stream. You have probably been thirstier but it is difficult to say, as you have to drink a lot during the day anyway because your job is physically demanding. You think you have lost about 3 kg in weight; you have always been a big eater and in spite of your job you have been putting on weight over the last five years until recently. You know you should probably lose some weight but you like your burgers, chips and beer. You do not smoke.

You are married with two children, no problems at home. You work for the council: park maintenance.

Last week the doctor wasn't sure what was wrong with you so he sent you for blood tests and urine tests and you have come back today for the results.

You have no other problems.

Past medical history

Appendicectomy age 22 years.

Family history

Father died age 75 years: heart attack.
Mother age 80 years alive and well.
Maternal grandmother: diabetes. You are not sure if she had injections or tablets, but you do know she was blind.

Ideas and concerns

It has crossed your mind that you might have diabetes but you are hoping it is something else . . . a water infection or maybe your prostate, maybe you are just working too hard. If the doctor tells you it is diabetes you will be upset, but not show this too obviously. You know that diabetes means you have to give up sweet things and that your lifestyle will be affected. You also believe that diabetes can make you go blind (your grandmother) and you will tell the doctor of your worries if you are asked about your concerns. You do not know that diabetes can affect your heart and kidneys. You are aware that raised cholesterol is not good for the heart.

If the doctor asks you if you have any questions you will ask about needing injections as you know that some people have these for diabetes. You will be happier if you are told you only need to diet or take tablets at the moment. You would also like to know if diabetes will affect your work. You drive a council van around the town.

Marking

The clinical observer gives the mark out of 30. The SP gives a mark out of 5. Tables 12.3–12.5 give examples of mark sheets for this scenario.

Table 12.3   Mark sheet: completed by clinical observer

Competency/behaviour	Excellent	Satisfactory	Not done or poor
1 Introduces self and ascertains reason for consultation (for test results)	2	1	0

Continued

Table 12.3 Continued

Competency/behaviour	Excellent	Satisfactory	Not done or poor
2 Discussion on diabetes:			
Explains result show type 2 diabetes	2	1	0
Determines what is already known	2		0
Explains what diabetes is	2	1	0
Explains risks of the condition: heart, circulation, kidneys, eyes	4	2	0
3 Discusses raised cholesterol:			
Advises it contributes to heart/circulation risks	2	1	0
Management by diet to start	2	1	0
4 Discussion of management:			
Explains need for diet and to lose weight	1	0.50	0
Explains need to check blood sugar regularly	1	0.50	0
Refers to nurse/diabetes educator	1	0.50	0
Explains management: diet to start, tablets if blood sugar remains high	2	1	0
5 Refers to dietician	1		0
6 Explores patient's concerns:			
Grandmother, blindness	2	1	0
Driving	2	1	0
7 Checks patient understanding of information presented	2	1	
8 Arranges follow-up (1–2 weeks)	2	1	0
Mark /30			

Table 12.4 Communication skills – process mark sheet: simulated patient

Did not introduce self, poor communication, much use of jargon, did not check your understanding, did not ask if you had any questions, no empathy, no interest in you. You would not want to see this doctor again	Did not introduce self, communication unsatisfactory, much use of jargon, did not check your understanding, did not ask if you had any questions, minimal empathy. You would not want to see this doctor again	Introduced self, adequate communication, some jargon, did not check your understanding, did not ask if you had any questions, minimal empathy. You would be reluctant to see this doctor again	Introduced self, satisfactory communication, with some jargon, checked you understood but only partial exploration of your concerns. Empathic. You would see this doctor again	Introduced self, good communication, minimal jargon, checked you understood, and explored your concerns. Empathic. You would see this doctor again	Introduced self. Excellent communication. Checked your understanding and explored your concerns in depth. Good information. Empathic. You would certainly see this doctor again
0	1	2	3	4	5

Table 12.5 Global mark at this station: consensus by observer and simulated patient

Poor performance		Neither poor nor good		Excellent performance	
0	1	2	3	4	5

Higher examinations

Membership examinations of the specialist royal colleges in the UK have a clinical component, often in the form of an OSCE. At present the membership examination of the Royal College of General Practitioners (MRCGP) requires candidates to submit a videotape of real consultations for assessment. Candidates who are unable to provide a video recording, may complete a simulated surgery, but numbers are restricted. The competencies that are assessed in the simulated surgery are shown in Box 12.5. In 2007 the MRCGP will include an OSCE. Stations for membership examinations are confidential but examples, together with marking guidelines and examiners' comments, are available on the relevant websites. Any of the scenarios in this book could be adapted as practice stations if marking sheets are developed in line with the appropriate college syllabus and competencies assessed.

Box 12.5 Competencies assessed in the simulated surgery for the MRCGP[21]

- Information gathering: interview/history taking (includes relevant biopsychosocial components)
- Awareness of patient's concerns (includes empathy)
- Communication/explanation
- Management options: agrees these with patient (involves patient in decision)
- Anticipatory care: implications for patient (includes health promotion and prevention)

Summary

There are several issues to consider when devising scenarios for assessment. The examiners must be clear as to what is being tested, how marks are awarded, the input of the SP and whether the candidate is to be given feedback. There are a variety of 'off-the-shelf' marking sheets, or one may be developed specifically for the scenario used.

References

1 Rethans J-J, Norcini JJ, Baron-Maldonado M *et al*. The relationship between competence and performance: implications for assessing practice performance. *Med Educ*. 2002; **36**: 901–9.
2 Miller GE. The assessment of clinical skills/competence/performance. *Acad Med*. 1990; **65** (Suppl): S63–7.
3 Wass V, van der Vleuten C, Shatzer J *et al*. Assessment of clinical competence. *Lancet*. 2001; **357**: 945–9.
4 Rethans JJ and Saebu L. Do general practitioners act consistently in real practice when they meet the same patient twice? Examination of intradoctor variation using standardized (simulated) patients. *BMJ*. 1997; **314**: 1170.
5 Harden RA and Gleeson FA. ASME medical educational booklet No 8: Assessment of medical competence using an objective structured clinical examination (OSCE). *J Med Educ*. 1979; **13**: 41–54.
6 Royal College of General Practitioners. *General Practice Workload. Information sheet No 3*. London: Royal College of General Practitioners, 2004.
7 Deveugle M, Derese A, Brink-Muinen A *et al*. Consultation length in general practice: cross sectional study in six European countries. *BMJ*. 2002; **325**: 472.
8 Wass V and Jolly B. Does observation add to the validity of the long case? *Med Educ*. 2001; **35**: 729–34.
9 Colliver JA, Willis MS, Robbs RS *et al*. Assessment of empathy in a standardized patient examination. *Teach Learn Med*. 1998; **10**: 8–11.

10 Allen J, Evans A, Foulkes J *et al*. Simulated surgery in the summative assessment of general practice training: results of a trial in the Trent and Yorkshire regions. *Br J Gen Pract*. 1998; **48**: 1219–23.

11 Kinnersley P and Pill R. Potential of using simulated patients to study the performance of general practitioners. *Br J Gen Pract*. 1993; **43**: 297–9.

12 Rethans J-J, Sturmans F, Drop R and van der Vleuten C. Assessment of the performance of general practitioners by the use of standardized (simulated) patients. *Br J Gen Pract*. 1991; **41**: 97–9.

13 Gorter SL, Rethans J-J, Scherpier AJJA *et al*. How to introduce incognito standardized patients into outpatient clinics of specialists in rheumatology. *Med Teach*. 2001; **23**: 138–44.

14 Van der Vleuten C and Swanson D. Assessment of clinical skills with standardized patients: state of the art. *Teach Learn Med*. 1990; **2**: 58–76.

15 Thistlethwaite JE. The use of incognito simulated patients in general practice: a feasibility study. *Education for Primary Care*. 2003; **14**: 419–25.

16 Neighbour R. Reflections on the ethics of assessment. *Education for Primary Care*. 2003; **14**: 406–10.

17 Reznic RK, Regehr G, Yee G *et al*. Process-rating forms versus task-specific checklists in an OSCE for medical licensure. *Acad Med*. 1998; **73**: S97–99.

18 Schwatz MH, Colliver JA, Bardes CL *et al*. Global ratings of videotaped performance versus global ratings of actions recorded in checklists: a criterion for performance assessment with standardized patients. *Acad Med*. 1999; **74**: 1028–32.

19 Angoff W. Scales, norms and equivalent scores. In: R Thorndike (ed). *Educational Measurement*. Washington DC: American Council on Education, 1971, pp 508–600.

20 Vu NV, Barrows H, Marcy M *et al*. Six years of comprehensive clinical performance based assessment using standardised patients at the Southern Illinois University School of Medicine. *Acad Med*. 1992; **62**: 42–50.

21 www.rcgp.org.uk/exam/modules/simsurgery/simsurg4.asp (accessed 9 February 2006).

Further reading on standard setting

• www.measurementresearch.com/media/standards.pdf (accessed 9 February 2006).
• Friedman B-D M. AMEE Guide No 18: Standard setting in student assessment. *Med Teach*. 2000; **22**: 120–30.

Chapter 13

Recent developments in communication skills training

This chapter explores:

- new developments in experiential learning using simulated patients
- the role of clinical teaching associates
- communication and clinical skills
- simulated patients and models
- overseas-trained doctors
- patients communicating with their doctors.

Because of the success of working with SPs to help students and qualified health professionals learn and develop their communication skills, medical educators (and SPs) are always thinking of new ways in which to enhance the role of SPs further in education. We have already explored the ways in which SPs work, give feedback and assess. In this chapter we look at other successful methods that capitalise on the tremendous power of the SP as an aid to learning, and think about possible developments in the future.

Clinical teaching associates

Clinical teaching associates (CTAs) are lay women from the community who are trained to provide teaching and feedback to health professionals and students about the technical and interpersonal skills required in intimate female examinations, while they (the CTAs) are being examined. The first reports of the development of a CTA training programme in the United States were published in the late 1970s, so this is not a new process.[1] However medical schools in the UK have been slow to introduce this method of teaching, with a team from Guys, Kings and Thomas's (GKT) Medical School in London writing about their first experiences of the method as late as 2003.[2] Now the practice is widespread. The CTAs help students learn about the pelvic, vaginal and breast examination of an asymptomatic woman, how to insert a speculum and how to obtain a cervical smear. In some medical schools male CTAs do similar instruction with regard to the male genitourinary system. (CTAs are also referred to as gynaecological teaching associates (GTAs) if they concentrate on the vaginal examination and taking cervical smears, rather than breast examination as well.)

CTAs are recruited in similar ways to other SPs. Interviews are vital and the women should be aware of exactly what it is they are learning to do. The necessary skills (after training) and attributes of CTAs are shown in Box 13.1. Training is given by an experienced clinician. After training, the novice CTA should be paired with an experienced CTA for several teaching sessions until the novice is completely comfortable with the procedure.

Not everyone who is suited to be an SP will be able to work as a CTA. While not strictly speaking 'simulated patients' the CTA programmes include the women teaching students about communication with their patients in relation to these intimate examinations. They also may give formative assessment of these skills and advise medical educators of any students who act inappropriately or who are too embarrassed to engage with the learning. Students who receive this type of training develop better skills than those who learn to perform intimate examinations 'on the job', i.e. in outpatient clinics, in general practice or in theatre (in these locations it is important to obtain informed consent from the patient first).

Box 13.1   Skills and attributes of CTAs

- Knowledge of normal female anatomy
- Ability to demonstrate the correct technique for breast and pelvic examinations
- Feeling comfortable being examined by clinical learners
- Patience and sensitivity
- Ability to give constructive feedback
- Excellent communication and interpersonal skills

Students attending CTA-run sessions may never have examined female genitalia before. Many students will be embarrassed; for some this embarrassment may take the form of making inappropriate remarks or being so anxious that they are unable to perform the examination; hence the need for sensitive and non-judgemental women, who are able to interact with students and recognise their anxieties, but who are also able to correct students' language. After the introductory session that may involve up to eight students, students work in pairs with two CTAs. CTAs never work alone. The learning outcomes for a session are shown in Box 13.2 and the outline of a typical learning experience in Box 13.3.

Box 13.2   Learning outcomes for the CTA session

- Being able to carry out a well woman check with sensitivity
- Awareness of a woman's perspective on intimate examinations
- Consideration of the need for a chaperone and who is appropriate for this
- Appropriate use of language before, during and after the examination
- Clinical skills of breast and pelvic examination
- Obtaining a cervical smear
- Awareness of cervical smear protocol and after care

Box 13.3   A CTA-led learning session

- Introduction: students and CTAs introduce themselves. Outline of learning outcomes and format of session. Discussion of any anxieties

---

Continued

- DVD: demonstration of breast and pelvic examinations
- Handling of different types of specula and spatulae for obtaining smears
- Demonstration: two CTAs run through the well woman check, with one taking the clinician's role, and the other the patient's role. Opportunity for students to ask questions
- Practical component: two CTAs and two students work together. Each student conducts a well woman check of one CTA, including interview, breast and pelvic examinations. The second CTA acts as chaperone/facilitator/instructor. Feedback from students and CTAs
- Debriefing: all students and CTAs come together to discuss the content and process. What further learning is needed?

While the practical component of the session concentrates on the examination of the asymptomatic woman, if there is time, or at another session, the students may also practise their gynaecological and sexual history taking with the CTA. From a theoretical point of view, it is not the role of the CTA to discuss the evidence for screening tests in asymptomatic women, in particular the merits of routine breast examination. Students need to learn breast examination and have the skill to distinguish between normal and abnormal breast tissue.

Scenarios for a CTA: gynaecological and sexual history from asymptomatic woman

CTA 1

'I am Brenda Howell, a 42-year-old librarian. I have come to see the doctor today for a routine cervical smear. It is three years since my last, which was normal. My periods are regular. I bleed for five days every four weeks. Occasionally I am a few days early or late. My last period was about two weeks ago. I have been married for 12 years to Peter. He had a vasectomy five years ago. We have two daughters aged ten and eight. Peter and I have sexual intercourse about once a week. It is rarely painful. I never bleed after sex and never bleed between periods. Sometimes I have a discharge but it is not offensive and clears up by itself. I had thrush about three months ago and treated myself.'

CTA 2 (if younger CTA available)

'I am Paula Cleveland, a 23-year-old secretary. I have come to see the doctor today for a cervical smear. I have never had a smear before and I am a bit anxious about it. I know what smears are for but I would be glad of some further explanation. What happens if I have something wrong? I have been on the contraceptive pill (Microgynon) since I was 16. My periods are regular with this. My last period was three weeks ago. Occasionally I have missed a pill, but this has never caused a problem . . . I have never missed more than one. I have had several sexual partners. I have been with my current boyfriend for six months. We use condoms usually, but not always. I am not particularly worried about sexually transmitted diseases, but I wouldn't mind having a test for them if the doctor suggests it.'

Scenario CTA 2 assesses the student's skill in running through the cervical smear process with a patient who has not had one before. Students should not use jargon and should check understanding.

Combining practising communication skills with clinical skills

The CTA programme is an example of experiential learning in which students combine practice in communication with developing a new clinical skill, i.e. breast and pelvic examination. Whenever students and qualified health professionals learn new skills, the communication aspects of such skills should also be explored. For example, when learning to suture, excise skin lesions or apply a plaster of Paris, the learner should think about how to explain the procedure to the patient before and during the task. If practising to start with on a model, the facilitator should remind learners that if this were a real patient, communication and explanation would be important.

Working with simulated patients and models

Roger Kneebone of Imperial College London has written extensively about clinical skills training, where clinical skills refers to the full package of eliciting a history, carrying out an examination, investigations, making a diagnosis, planning management, communication and professionalism. He and his team have developed a method of combining the experience of working with simulated patients and procedural skills development with bench top models.[3,4] For example, a student is learning to take blood from a patient. The student first practises on a model arm. Once the student is proficient in obtaining blood, the model arm becomes one of the arms of an SP (the real arm is concealed beneath a blanket). The student now interacts with the patient as he/she takes blood. The student has to explain the procedure, check the patient is comfortable and ensure correct follow-up. After this process, the student may graduate to taking blood from real patients in clinical settings.

This process moves away from the artificiality of students introducing themselves to models: a one-way communication flow. The SP is able to respond and later give feedback. The clinical tutor also gives feedback. For examinations SPs again lend authenticity to situations. Candidates may be asked to examine a patient's breasts. A model is used but the simulated patient can comment on the interaction, as if she were being examined.

Experiential learning sessions for doctors whose first language is not English (overseas-trained doctors/ international medical graduates)

Many countries are currently experiencing a shortage of doctors and are recruiting clinicians from overseas. Often these doctors speak English as their second or even third language, and while they may have a good grasp of technical medical jargon, their idiom and 'street language' hampers their ability to communicate with patients. Running learning sessions with SPs and these doctors is an excellent way of helping them develop not only language skills, but also consultation skills. In their own countries there may not have been a climate of patient partnership and shared decision making. Depending on their country of origin and their registration status, some of these doctors may already be working in the UK at the time of this training. They should therefore be able to bring cases from their experience to work through and discuss.

Suggested training course for overseas-trained doctors

Our suggestion is to offer four half-day sessions for up to six participants, working in groups of three to six. There would be one session a week and they would be delivered at a fixed, well-resourced venue on consecutive weeks. Two SPs would be needed, with several scripted roles, as well as two facilitators, depending on group size (*see* Box 13.4).

Participants would be invited to consider topics and problems in communication such as:

- basic consultation skills
- defining and exploring the patient's agenda and concerns
- exploring and managing cross-cultural attitudes to medical treatments and prescriptions
- working with colleagues and other health professionals.

Participants would also be expected to define their own objectives regarding communication, based on their experiences of working in a new country.

Part of the preparation for the workshops would involve the facilitators exploring the views of patients with respect to consulting with overseas doctors, in order to prepare sensitive and appropriate SP scenarios.

Box 13.4   Aims of course for overseas-trained doctors

- To create a safe learning environment
- To improve participants' communication and cross-cultural skills
- To address participants' personal communication problems
- To prepare for any forthcoming examinations
- To improve patients' outcomes in future consultations with course participants

---

Methods to be used

- *Suitable group building exercises* would be carried out, and a safe learning environment developed.
- *Video analysis*: an example of a good consultation between a doctor and a patient would be shown to the group. This may be an actual consultation or use an SP scenario. A discussion of the components of the interview would follow, with feedback following Pendleton's guidelines.[5]
- The relationship between the process and content of the consultation would be determined, and how a good medical knowledge does not necessarily translate into effective communication skills. The importance of good communication skills in achieving a satisfactory outcome for the patient, including shared decision making, would be demonstrated.

- Members of the group would conduct a *simulated interview* using a scripted role. Participants would receive feedback on their performance. Group discussion would be facilitated to draw out salient points relating to communication and cross-cultural issues.
- *Further simulated roles would be developed by the group* based on individual learning needs. These new roles would be enacted by the simulated patients followed by further feedback.

An outline of the course is shown in Table 13.1.

Table 13.1 Timetable for overseas doctors' workshop (timings are flexible and are given as illustration only)

Time	Session 1	Session 2	Session 3	Session 4
08.45–09.00	Registration	Registration	Registration	Registration
09.00–09.30	Introductions	Two groups of four prepared scenarios Revision of feedback	Components of a good interview	Client-based scenarios
	Group formation SPs work on roles			
09.30–10.15	Course outline and discussion	First SP role	Client-based scenarios with optional prepared roles	Client-based scenarios
	Setting of personal objectives Brainstorm: communication skills			
Break				
10.30–11.15	'Rules' of feedback Videotape analysis and feedback	Second SP role	Prepared role	Mini-OSCE
11.15–12.00	First SP role	Third SP role	Prepared role	Mini-OSCE
12.00–12.30	Discussion	Whole-group feedback	Whole-group feedback	Evaluation
12.30	Close	Close	Close	Close

Session 1

Objectives

- To create a safe learning environment.
- To introduce participants to experiential learning methods.
- To develop language and ideas used in skilled communication.
- To observe an example of good communication.
- To experience an SP interview.
- To give and receive feedback on communication skills.

The day starts with an icebreaker – all present respond to who they are and where they are from. The facilitator stresses that the sessions are confidential and the aim is to improve our communication skills. Small-group work identifies the ideas of content, process and perception, of a patient interview. Group work is flip-charted. A videotape of a doctor–patient interview (preferably a doctor who is or will be working with the group) is shown and discussed using Pendleton's rules of feedback.[5] One or two participants practise their own skills using an SP and a prepared scenario. The interviewer receives feedback.

Session 2

Objectives

- To continue to build a safe learning environment.
- To experience an SP interview with feedback.
- To develop communication skills.

This session starts with individuals considering what their hopes and concerns are with respect to the course. The larger group is split into groups of three to four. Three participants undertake an SP interview with feedback given as appropriate. The whole group meets to discuss key points. Participants are requested to bring a personally challenging patient scenario to work with in the next session.

Session 3

Objectives

- To discuss in detail the components of a good interview.
- To address individual learning needs.

Participants discuss their understanding of the structure of a patient interview. Typical components are *building rapport, finding out* the patient's problem, *explaining* the patient's management and *sharing decisions*, and *closing* the interview. In pairs, participants discuss one component, considering what it means to both doctor and patient. This is reported back to the whole group.

Participants work with an SP using a scenario which they help to generate and which is based on a challenging situation they wish to explore.

Session 4

Objectives

- To focus on participants' learning needs.
- To offer experience of OSCE-type examinations.
- To evaluate the course.

Participants continue working with SPs using a mix of prepared and suggested roles. There is a mini-OSCE with marking and feedback. Participants complete a course evaluation form.

Developing communication skills for patients

This book has concentrated on experiential learning for health professionals and students in order to help them improve their communication with patients. There is no reason why such techniques could not be employed with patients to help them gain maximum benefit from their clinical interactions. Patients (or clients) in self-help groups, patient participation groups or from other sources, would come together to work with simulated clinicians and facilitators. As Dr Muir Gray (director of the UK National Screening Committee) has written: '. . . every medical curriculum now includes communication and patient consultation skills at its core. However, it is not the clinician who consults, it is the patient, so surely it is also the patient who needs help to develop these skills'.[6]

For example, Towle and Godolpin from Vancouver have devised a list of competencies that patients require to be able to participate fully in shared decision making with their doctors (*see* Box 13.5).[7] How are patients to learn such skills? One way is practice in simulated consultations.

Box 13.5   Competencies for patients for informed shared decision making[6]

- Define (for oneself) the preferred doctor–patient relationship
- Find a physician and establish, develop, and adapt a partnership
- Articulate (for oneself) health problems, feelings, beliefs and expectations in an objective and systematic manner
- Communicate with the physician in order to understand and share relevant information clearly and at the appropriate time in the medical interview
- Access information
- Evaluate information
- Negotiate decisions, give feedback, resolve conflict, agree on an action plan

---

Summary

The possibilities of simulation, working with simulated patients, clinicians and teams, are boundless. We have touched on many types of learning situations, from our own experience and that of our colleagues. There are as many scenarios as patient–professional interactions. We have learnt from real and simulated patients. An important message indeed is not to forget the patient in devising roles and situations, to strive for authenticity and take note of the evaluation.

References

1   Kretzschmar RUM. Evolution of the gynaecology teaching associate: an education specialist. *Am J Obstet Gynecol*. 1978; **131**: 367–73.
2   Pickard S, Baraitser P, Rymer J *et al*. Can gynaecology teaching associates provide high quality effective training for medical students in the United Kingdom? Comparative study. *BMJ*. 2003; **327**: 389–92.
3   Kneebone RL, Kidd J, Nestel D *et al*. An innovative model for teaching and learning clinical procedures. *Med Educ*. 2002; **36**: 628–34.
4   Kneebone RL and Nestel D. Learning clinical skills – the place of simulation and feedback. *Clin Teach*. 2005; **2**: 86–90.
5   Pendleton D, Schofield T, Tate P and Havelock P. *The Consultation: an approach to learning and teaching*. Oxford: Oxford University Press, 1984.
6   Muir Gray JA. *The Resourceful Patient*. Oxford: eRosetta Press, 2002.
7   Towle A and Godolphin W. Framework for teaching and learning informed shared decision-making. *BMJ*. 1999; **319**: 766–71.

Index